Prefix
MTW

0009504

Prefix

D1758905

GERIATRIC

DERMATOLOGY

957.32
m

GERIATRIC
DERMATOLOGY

Edited by
Robert A. Norman

Department of Dermatology
Nova Southeastern University, Florida
and
President and CEO
Dermatology Healthcare, Florida

LIBRARY
PEMBURY HOSPITAL
01892 823535

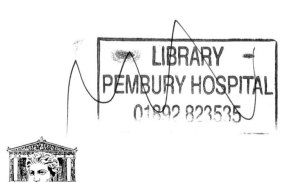

The Parthenon Publishing Group
International Publishers in Medicine, Science & Technology

NEW YORK   LONDON

Library of Congress Cataloging-in-Publication Data

Geriatric dermatology / edited by Robert A. Norman.

    p. ; cm.

   Includes bibliographical references and index.

   ISBN I-85070-311-6 (alk.paper)

   1. Geriatric dermatology. 2. Skin--Diseases--Age factors. 3. Skin--Aging. I. Norman, Robert A., 1955-

   [DNLM: 1. Skin Diseases--therapy--Aged. WR 650 G369 2001]

RL73.A35 G465 2001

618.97′65--dc21

                        00-052879

British Library Cataloguing in Publication Data

Geriatric dermatology

   1. Geriatric dermatology

   2. Skin--Diseases--Treatment

   I. Norman, Robert A.

   618.9′765

   ISBN 1850703116

Published in the USA by
The Parthenon Publishing Group Inc.
One Blue Hill Plaza
PO Box 1564, Pearl River
NY 10965, USA

Published in the UK and Europe by
The Parthenon Publishing Group Limited
Casterton Hall, Carnforth
Lancs., LA6 2LA, UK

Copyright © 2001
The Parthenon Publishing Group

No part of this book may be reproduced in any form without permission from the publishers, except for the quotation of brief passages for the purposes of review.

Typeset by Siva Math Setters, Chennai, India
Printed by T. G. Hostench S.A., Spain

Contents

List of contributors

A. R. Ahmed
Department of Oral Medicine
  and Diagnostic Sciences
Harvard School of Dental Medicine
188 Longwood Avenue
Boston, MA 02115

M. Alam
Department of Dermatology
Columbia University
161 Fort Washington Avenue
New York, NY 10032

Y. M. Bello
University of Miami School of Medicine
Department of Dermatology
  and Cutaneous Surgery
PO Box 016250
Miami, FL 33101

B. P. Glick
South Florida Skin and Laser Center
5901 Colonial Drive, Suite 106
Margate, FL 33063

J. Z. Litt
Case Western Reserve
  University School of Medicine
Cleveland, OH

S. L. Moschella
Department of Dermatology
Lahey Clinic
41 Mall Road
Burlington, MA 01805

R. A. Norman
Department of Dermatology
Nova Southeastern University
Tampa, FL 33615

T. J. Phillips
Department of Dermatology
Boston Medical Center
609 Albany Street
Boston, MA 02118

G. Rebell
Greater Miami Skin and Laser Center
Mt. Sinai Medical Center
Miami Beach, FL

J. L. Roberts
Northwest Cutaneous Research Specialists
Department of Dermatology
Oregon Health Sciences University
2222 Northwest Lovejoy, Suite 419
Portland, OR 97210

A. I. Rojas
University of Connecticut Health Center
Department of Medicine
263 Farmington Avenue
Farmington, CT 06030

N. Sami
Department of Oral Medicine
  and Diagnostic Sciences
Harvard School of Dental Medicine
188 Longwood Avenue
Boston, MA 02115

R. K. Scher
Department of Dermatology
College of Physicians and Surgeons
Columbia University
New York, NY 10032

P. I. Schneiderman
Department of Dermatology
College of Physicians and Surgeons
Columbia University
New York, NY 10032

S. P. Stone
Division of Dermatology
Southern Illinois University
   School of Medicine
PO Box 19644
Springfield, IL 62794–9644

R. Townsend
Southern Regional Area Health Education
   Consortium (SRAHEC)
1601 Owen Drive
Fayetteville, NC 28305

M. Zaiac
Greater Miami Skin and Laser Center
Mt. Sinai Medical Center
Miami Beach, FL

N. Zaias
Department of Dermatology
Mt. Sinai Medical Center
Miami Beach, FL

Preface

The purpose of *Geriatric Dermatology* is to provide an overview of the diagnosis and treatment of geriatric skin diseases for those working in the fields of dermatology, primary care, geriatrics, and other areas of medicine involving care of the elderly. The text begins with a general overview of the aging of the world's population, and the major dermatological problems that may arise in elderly patients in long-term/nursing home care.

The book draws together a panel of experts in geriatric dermatology, who contribute chapters on many of the topics of major importance to this field. In order to facilitate the diagnosis of geriatric skin diseases, there is a summary of the dermatological disorders that are frequently encountered in the elderly, including eczematous dermatitis, skin infections and neoplasias. This is followed by a description of the most common geriatric hair and scalp disorders, including graying, alopecia and scalp psoriasis. The book also provides comprehensive coverage of the diagnosis and treatment of leg, foot, and nail diseases – the second most common site of skin complaints in the elderly after the face. Treatment of superficial mycoses (fungal infections) is described in detail, as is management of scabies and pediculosis. In addition, the book addresses less common geriatric conditions such as blistering diseases. The major adverse drug reactions on the skin are outlined; these are frequently encountered in the elderly because many are taking multiple medications. Leg ulcers are also covered, a frequent problem owing to venous insufficiency, arterial disease and diabetic nephropathy. Diabetes is more prevalent in the elderly population, and the book concludes with a description of the diagnosis and treatment of diabetic complications of dermatology, such as scleroderma and dermopathy.

The study of diseases that impact on the elderly population is a crucial and growing area of interest in medicine. While this book is not intended to provide encyclopedic coverage of dermatological syndromes, many of the diseases of major importance in the field of geriatric dermatology have been included. As the world's population ages, this text will provide a timely addition to the field of geriatric medicine.

R. A. Norman

Dedication

To the many practitioners who provide dermatology care for the elderly

To my students

To the many physicians who have helped me along the way, I give my heartfelt thanks, especially Dr Erwin Gutowitz, Dr Jeffrey Holtzman, Dr Richard Brown, and Dr Richard Miller

To my wife and children

The aging of the world's population

1

R. A. Norman

INTRODUCTION

Over the past few years the world's population has continued on its remarkable transition path from a state of high birth and death rates to one characterized by low birth and death rates. At the heart of that transition has been the growth in the number and proportion of older persons. The size of the world's elderly population has been growing for centuries; what is new is its current rapid acceleration. The increase in the 60-and-over population in the industrialized nations of Europe and North America has generally outpaced total population growth in recent decades. Such a rapid, large and ubiquitous growth has never been seen in the history of civilization (www.un.org; www.who.org; www.popin.org).

The current demographic revolution is predicted to continue well into the coming centuries. Its major features include the following:

(1) One of every ten persons is now aged 60 years or older; by 2050, one out of five will be 60 years or older; and by 2150, one out of three persons will be 60 years or older.

(2) The older population itself is aging. The number of very old people (aged 80+ years) is projected to grow by a factor of from 8 to 10 times on the global scale, between 1950 and 2050. By 2150, about a third of the older population will be 80 years or older.

(3) The majority of older persons (55%) are women. Among the oldest old (85 years or older), 65% are women.

(4) Striking differences exist between regions. One out of five Europeans, but one out of twenty Africans, is aged 60 years or older.

(5) As the tempo of aging in developing countries is more rapid than in developed countries, developing countries will have less time than the developed countries to adapt to the consequences of an aging population.

(6) By the end of year 2000, the majority of the world's older persons (51%) will be living in urban areas. It is projected that by the end of the year 2000, almost 78% of older women and more than 75% of older men in more developed regions will be living in urban areas. The majority of older persons of both sexes in developing regions are expected to remain in rural areas[1,2].

The number of elderly is expected soon to increase steeply, with implications for a vast increase in the numbers of persons requiring special services (health, recreation, housing, nutrition, etc.) There must be a recognition of the possible implications of an aging society for the whole range of social institutions, from education and family to business and government. It is well known that the number of people aged over 80 is set to increase dramatically this century. It is less appreciated, however, that this demographic change will be most significant in less developed countries. The world's population aged 60 and over increased by more than 12 million in 1995, 80% of this increase occurring in less-developed countries, and this trend is expected to continue in the future. For example, over the next 50 years the elderly population is projected to increase by 23% in the UK, but by 292% in Brazil, 324% in Mexico and 414% in Indonesia. Poorer and less developed countries are in the main totally unprepared for this phenomenon, and their problems will be exacerbated by social change, including urbanization with breakdown of family support, a trend towards nuclear families, work outside the home for women, and (to some extent) a change in the traditional values of reverence for older people (www.un.org; www.who.org; www.popin.org).

A CASE STUDY – JAPAN

No other population in the world is aging as quickly as that of Japan. By the year 2020, according to Japan's Institute for Population Problems, an organ of the Ministry of Health and Welfare, people aged 65 and over will account for 25.5% of the nation's population; this will be more than double the 12.1% of 1990. Because elderly Japanese have the longest life spans among any developed nation in the world, daily care for many infirm people can last 10 years or more. This places great stress on both professional care-givers and the bedridden person's family.

In Japan, unlike the US and many European countries, an individual's health care continues to be covered completely by social insurance, no matter how old the person is, and in the fiscal year 1995 various union and government health insurance plans covered about 71 million Japanese. But even though most Japanese are covered by medical insurance, a severe imbalance is putting enormous financial pressure on this system (www.un.org; www.who.org; www.popin.org).

FEMALE ADVANTAGE IN LIFE EXPECTANCY PARTIALLY OFFSET BY DISABILITY

As life expectancy at birth and at older ages increases, the quality of that longer life becomes a major issue. The concept of healthy life expectancy (also called active life expectancy or disability-free life expectancy) refers to the average number of years that persons may expect to be free of limitations of function due to one or more chronic disease conditions. It is difficult to precisely compare measures of healthy life expectancy among nations because of computational and conceptual differences.

Various studies show that women who reach 65 can expect to live more disability-free years than their male counterparts (except in the Netherlands). However, because women have higher life expectancy than do men at age 65, the proportion of disability-free remaining life at age 65 tends to be greater for men.

THE OLDEST OLD

In many countries of the world, the oldest old (those 85 years and older) are the fastest growing portion of the elderly population. The oldest old constituted 23% of the world's 60-and-over population in 1996, 30% in more-developed countries and 19% in less-developed countries. More than 43% of the world's oldest old in 1996 lived in just four countries: the People's Republic of China, the United States, India and Japan. In some African and Asian nations the population age 75 and over at present constitutes less than 1% of the total population. This contrasts sharply with the situation in Europe and North America, where the proportion of the oldest old reaches as high as 8.5% (Sweden). The numerical growth and increasing heterogeneity of the oldest old challenge social planners to seek further information about this group, since the oldest old consume disproportionate amounts of health and long-term care services.

The growth in the number of the oldest old (aged 85 and over) is of great public concern. During 1995 to 2010, this population is expected to grow by 56%, as compared with 13% for the populations aged 65 to 84. In subsequent decades, especially between 2030 and 2050, the 85-and-over age group will grow sharply as the 'baby-boom' cohorts age. The 85-and-over age group is expected to increase from 3.6 million in 1995 to 5.7 million in 2010, to 8.5 million in 2030, and to 18.2 million in 2050. Thus, while the expected increase from 2010 to 2030 is just less than 50%, the increase from 2030 to 2050 is 114%. The cumulative growth in the 85-and-over population from 1995 to 2050 is anticipated to be more than 400%, and the proportion of that group in the total population is likely to increase from 1.4% in 1995 to 4.6% in 2050.

Changes in the proportion of elderly in the total population have a different causal basis. The projections of a very high and increasing proportion of elderly from 2010 to 2030 are accounted for by three factors: (1) declining and low fertility in the past and the prospect of continuing low fertility up to 2030 (and beyond); (2) maturing of the baby-boom cohorts; and (3) sharp declines in mortality at the adult and older ages in the recent past and the prospect of continuing low mortality up to 2030 (and beyond). Once the baby-boom influx is over (i.e., has completely passed age 65) in 2030, the proportion of elderly in the total population is expected to stabilize[3].

The figures for all race groups combined tend to reflect mainly the changes in the white elderly population. Blacks, Asian and Pacific Islanders and Hispanics will share in the main trends described, but to a more intensive degree. Between 2010 and 2030, the size of these racial/ethnic groups will increase dramatically. Similarly, dramatic increases are projected between 2030 and 2050 for the 85-and-over age group in these populations. The rates of growth for Asian and Pacific Islanders (the main component of the 'other races' group) and Hispanics far exceed those for whites in all periods[4].

References

1. Manton KG, Liu K. The future growth of the long-term care populations: projections based on the 1977 National Nursing Home Survey and the 1982 Long-Term Care Survey. Presented at the *Third National Leadership Conference on Long-Term Care Issues*, Washington, DC, March 1984
2. Kunkel SR, Applebaum RA. Estimating the prevalence of long-term disability for an aging society. *J Gerontol: Social Sciences* 1992;475: S253–S260
3. Zedlewski SR, Barnes RO, Burt MK, *et al. The Needs of the Elderly in the 21st Century.* Washington, DC: Urban Institute, 1989
4. US Bureau of the Census. Population projections of the United States by age, sex, race, and Hispanic origin: 1995 to 2050. *Curr Pop Reports.* Washington, DC: US Government Printing Office, 1996a:25–1130

Dermatological problems and treatment in long-term/nursing-home care

2

R. A. Norman

INTRODUCTION

There is a growing need for expertise in dermatological consultations in the long-term care setting throughout the world. For example, in the United States Florida has the highest percentage of seniors, with 19% of its residents aged 65 and over; by 2020, this is expected to rise to 25.6%. For many people, the nursing home will be their final home. Others may remain in a nursing home for a short time as they recuperate from an illness or operation. About 20% of nursing-home residents are able to go home after a period of rehabilitation, therefore they may become part of an office-based practice[1].

Common skin problems in nursing-home care

Many of the same problems are seen in nursing homes as in an office practice. However, many studies have demonstrated that skin disease is more common in the geriatric population than in the general population, hence there is an increased frequency of certain diseases in nursing-home patients (Appendix 1). A large number of patients have miliaria, eczematous disorders, stasis dermatitis, chronic fungal disease, scabies, skin tears, ulcers and other maladies of immobility and chronicity. One study revealed that 40% of Americans between the ages of 65 and 74 years of age had a cutaneous disease significant enough to warrant treatment by a physician. Patients older than 74 years are even more likely to develop significant skin diseases[2,3].

Skin care in the elderly and disabled is a major challenge. Since most of the conditions encountered are dealt with in other chapters of this book, this chapter will concentrate on wound care with special reference to those in a nursing home suffering from ulcers – particularly pressure ulcers.

Chronic vs. acute wounds

A chronic wound is defined as a loss in tissue integrity produced by insult or injury that is of extended duration or frequent recurrence. An acute wound is one in which simple medical or surgical intervention produces a resolution.

Although in some animals – such as the toad – amputation of a limb can result in the regeneration of a new one identical to the original, in man only hepatic and epithelial tissues are capable of regeneration, and wound healing occurs by repair. In man, wounding that injures the dermis signals the body to restore the structural integrity via the synthesis of new tissue different from that originally present. The type of wound and mechanism by which the wound is closed depend on the extent of injury and the type of tissue injured. In chronic wounds, the healing time is longer and can be phased using markers such as the Clark model. Clark categorized healing into three phases: inflammation (from the moment of injury to approximately four to six days post injury); granulation tissue production (days 4 to 21); and matrix formation and remodeling (from 3 weeks to up to 2 years). Key cells in phase one include platelets, neutrophils, lymphocytes and epithelial cells. Macrophages play a crucial role in all three phases, and fibroblasts are important in phases 2 and 3. Superficial wounds, where only the epidermis or dermis is injured (partial thickness wounds) may heal rapidly via the process of re-epithelialization. Epithelial cells migrate toward one another from the edges of the wound, from the hair follicles, sebaceous glands and sweat glands, and eventually close the wound[2,4].

Wound recurrence factors

Chronic wounds often result from surgical procedures, traumatic insults, or metabolic, infectious, or neoplastic disorders. Pressure ulcers, diabetic ulcers, lower-leg ulcers, vascular ulcers, postoperative open wounds and enterocutaneous fistulae are frequent types of chronic wound[5].

Non-healing wounds generally occur in older individuals with multi-system problems, poor medical care and inadequate health habits. Chronic wounds often arise as a result of diabetes, cancer, liver, renal, or gastrointestinal illness. Radiation trauma victims, transplant patients and burn patients often suffer from chronic wounds. Drug therapy such as steroids can make a person more prone to wound development. Obesity, smoking, poor nutrition and immobility can delay wound repair. Given the many factors that predispose the older patient to chronic wound development, it is obviously crucial for any physician or care-giver to carefully assess their patients and work on preventive strategies such as weight control, smoking cessation, proper nutrition and appropriate drug usage. Wounds represent an enormous burden to the patient's economic and psychological well-being. The prevalence of chronic non-healing wounds can only be estimated. In 1989 in the United States, approximately 2 100 000 people had pressure ulcers, 3 000 000 had diabetic ulcers, 500 000 had vascular ulcers and 6500 had open wounds or fistulae, giving a total of some 5 606 500; the cost of healing a single pressure ulcer can range from $400 to $40 000[6].

Pressure ulcers

A pressure ulcer is a localized area of trauma or tissue necrosis resulting from lack of blood supply to the tissues involved (Figure 1). Although many factors contribute to the development of pressure ulcers, the four most critical are pressure, shearing forces, friction and moisture. Pressure results in ischemia and tissue damage. Shearing forces occur when layers of tissue slide on each other and twisting and stretching of blood vessels result in subsequent ischemia and damage. Friction is the force created when two surfaces in contact move across each other, for example when a patient is pulled across the bed sheets, thus eliminating the outer protective stratum corneum and accelerating the ulcerative process. Moisture from urine, feces, wound exudate, or perspiration leads to skin maceration and an increased risk of ulceration.

The vast majority of pressure ulcers occur on bony prominences in the lower part of the body, with the sacral and coccygeal areas, ischial tuberosities and greater trochanters accounting for the majority of sites. Other areas that are frequently involved include the fibular head, malleolus, heel and the medial condyle of the tibia. There are many consequences of pressure ulcers, some of which are life-threatening. Ulcers can be a source of sepsis and osteomyelitis, pyarthrosis, joint disarticulation and systemic amyloidosis.

Pressure ulcers have been categorized into four stages by the Agency for Health Care Policy and Research (AHCPR) (Table 1 and Figures 2 and 3).

Incidence and prevalence

High-risk populations include quadriplegics, critical care patients, the elderly (especially those with femoral fractures), persons with terminal cancer, end-stage renal, liver or heart disease, diabetics and those who are immunosuppressed; other risk factors include immobility, poor nutritional state, incontinence and altered levels of consciousness[7].

Table 1 Stages of pressure ulcers (Agency for Health Care Policy and Research guidelines)

Stage	Description
Stage I	Nonblanchable erythema of intact skin, the heralding lesion of skin ulceration. In individuals with darker skin, discoloration of the skin, warmth, edema, induration, or hardness may also be indicators
Stage II	Partial loss of the thickness of the skin involving the epidermis and/or dermis. The ulcer is superficial and presents clinically as an abrasion, blister, or shallow crater
Stage III	Full thickness skin loss involving damage or necrosis of subcutaneous tissue that may extend down to, but not through, underlying fascia. The ulcer presents clinically as a deep crater with or without undermining of adjacent tissue
Stage IV	Full thickness skin loss with extensive destruction, tissue necrosis, or damage to muscle, bone, or supporting structures (for example, tendon or joint capsule). Undermining and sinus tracts may also be associated with this stage

Table modified from: Panel on the Prediction and Prevention of Pressure Ulcers in Adults. *Pressure Ulcers in Adults: Prediction and Prevention. Quick Reference Guide for Clinicians*. AHCPR Publication No. 92-0050. Rockville, MD: Agency for Health Care Policy and Research, Public Health Service, US Department of Health and Human Services. May 1992

Risk assessment

Assessment of risk must be ongoing and holistic in nature; the information to be obtained should include:

(1) Establishment of baseline functional status including gait, falls, activities of daily living (ADL) abilities, hearing, vision and cognition;

(2) Nutritional assessment;

(3) Use of medications;

(4) Specific problems with regard to bowel or bladder incontinence; and

(5) Psychological assessment.

Prevention

The occurrence of pressure ulcers can be minimized by taking the following precautions:

(1) Mobility can be maximized by:
  (a) Avoiding prolonged bed rest and its adverse effects as far as possible;
  (b) Avoiding the use of restraints as much as possible; they do not protect patients and can lead to multiple problems including all the problems of immobility;
  (c) Involving rehabilitation specialists such as physical therapists and occupational therapists early on; and
  (d) Preventing contractures.

(2) Adequate nutrition can be ensured by:
  (a) Assessing nutrition including regular monitoring of intake, weight and appropriate laboratory parameters. Problems with anorexia should be assessed, including possible etiologies such as undiagnosed illness, depression, or other psychological problems, sensory loss or difficulty in swallowing;
  (b) Preventing deterioration in nutritional status, which can worsen rapidly in those who are marginally nourished to start with. Minimize days with NPO status and if prolonged consider alternative forms of nutritional support;
  (c) Utilizing supplements as appropriate;
  (d) Assuring a pleasant mealtime environment;
  (e) Providing adequate assistance with meals; and
  (f) Not overly restricting diet[8,9].

Bowel and bladder incontinence should be assessed and attempts made to treat them; they should not be accepted without a thorough evaluation as to the etiology of the problem and a trial of treatment strategies.

It is possible to protect against the adverse effects of external forces such as pressure, friction and shear by the following strategies:

(1) Utilizing proper positioning techniques and repositioning schedules, bearing in

mind that elevating the head of the bed produces shearing forces;

(2) Preventing shearing injuries by utilizing lifting devices to move patients and using lubricants, protective dressings or films and protective padding to reduce the incidence and extent of friction injuries;

(3) Utilizing the appropriate pressure-reducing devices for patients deemed to be at risk of contracting pressure ulcers;

(4) Utilizing appropriate skin care techniques, avoiding harsh cleansing products, excessively hot water and vigorous massage; and

(5) Providing a careful skin inspection at least daily for patients at risk, paying close attention to the heels as these are particularly at risk.

Healing

There are three processes involved in wound healing:

(1) Epithelial proliferation
(2) Granulation
(3) Wound contraction

Clinical care of pressure ulcers

The following factors should be considered in the initial treatment of ulcers:

(1) Saline irrigation provides a safe and appropriate cleansing method for most pressure ulcers. Agents toxic to wound tissue – such as povidone iodine, iodophor, sodium hypochlorite solution, hydrogen peroxide, or acetic acid – should not be used.

(2) Any necrotic tissue observed during wound assessment should be debrided if appropriate; all infected ulcers should be debrided rapidly, bearing in mind the need for pain control and adequate preparation of the patient. The most rapid method of removing areas of thick, adherent eschar and devitalized tissue is with sharp debridement generally utilizing sterile surgical scissors. Mechanical debridement involves wet-to-dry dressings, hydrotherapy and wound irrigation. Enzymatic debridement, utilizing topical debriding agents on devitalized tissues, should be considered when the patient cannot tolerate surgery and in non-infected ulcers. Autolytic debridement involves the use of a synthetic dressing over an ulcer, allowing the eschar to self-digest through the action of enzymes normally present in the wound fluid. It is not indicated for infected ulcers. Curetting the borders of the lesions often stimulates increased granulation and wound healing.

(3) All stage II, III and IV ulcers are colonized by bacteria and this colonization should be minimized through effective wound cleansing and debridement. Swab cultures only detect surface colonization and should not be used. Needle aspiration or biopsy can be used when a culture is needed. A biopsy is recommended to rule out malignancy with any chronic ulcer that is not healing by conventional measures, and a two-week trial of topical antibiotics (triple antibiotic, silver sulfadiazine) should be considered if a clean ulcer is not healing or continues to have exudate despite optimal care for two to four weeks. Impaired healing is encountered with high bacterial counts or osteomyelitis. Systemic antibiotics are appropriate for patients with bacteremia, sepsis, advancing cellulitis, or osteomyelitis, but not for local pressure ulcers. Cultures with Gram stains should be taken before the institution of any antibiotic therapy for infected wounds.

(4) Conservative measures such as support stockings, elevation of the legs and so-called 'bunny boots' or other devices should be used for protection whenever indicated, but aggressive care should be given to those patients with pronounced edema, signs of vascular compromise,

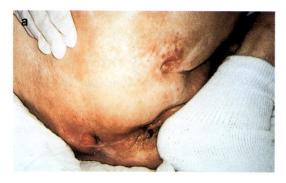

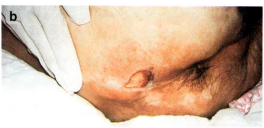

Figure 1   (a and b) Stage II and Stage III pressure ulcers

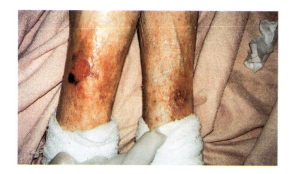

Figure 2   Stage II ulcers of lower extremities in a patient with stasis dermatitis

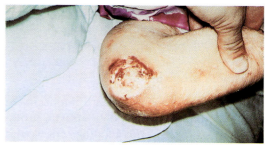

Figure 3   Non-healing pressure ulcer of elbow

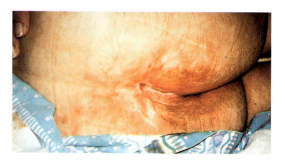

Figure 4   Healing sacral pressure ulcer

gangrene and diabetic and other troublesome ulcers. A consultation with a vascular surgeon may be indicated in such cases.

(5) Patients with contractures may benefit from treatment by a physical therapist, and podiatrists should be utilized for routine care and maintenance of the feet.

During treatment of all stages of pressure ulcers the following guidelines should be followed:

(1) Reduce pressure of the overlay of the bed, chair and on the heels (by means of pillows for example);

(2) Ensure adequate incontinence care q a.m. and PRN following each episode of incontinence;

(3) Reposition the patient every two hours, using a lift sheet and avoiding pressure to affected areas; ensure that he/she is out of bed and in a chair for not more than two hours at a time;

(4) Use pillows for positioning and avoid skin-on-skin contact or pressure;

(5) Obtain dietary consultation;

(6) Encourage intake of fluids, unless restricted;

(7) Have appropriate laboratory tests carried out – total protein and serum albumin, complete blood count (CBC) with differential, and zinc (if not previously obtained);

(8) Evaluate the area of wounding at each treatment application; and

(9) Document the area of wounding weekly and PRN if the wound heals or if the condition worsens[10].

Treatment protocols

Zinc and vitamins A and K are important in the comprehensive wound treatment protocol. Vitamin C, an antioxidant, speeds wound healing.

Stage I treatment protocol

(1) If the wound is on an extremity:
   (a) Cleanse with normal saline or commercial cleanser;
   (b) Apply protective ointment;
   (c) Apply foot splint, foot pillow, or elevate heels off bed with pillows.

Or:
   (a) Cleanse with normal saline or commercial cleanser;
   (b) Apply a skin prepping solution;
   (c) Cover with a transparent dressing;
   (d) Change every 5–7 days – frequency must be specific but individualized.

(2) If the wound is on the buttocks:
   (a) Cleanse entire buttocks and surrounding area with a no-rinse cleansing spray and pat dry;
   (b) Apply a second generation barrier cream;
   (c) Recleanse and reapply cream every shift. It is not necessary to remove all the old barrier cream with each cleansing, merely remove urine/feces or soiling before reapplying.

Stage II treatment protocol

Wound cleansing: flush the wound with normal saline or commercial wound cleanser. Dry the surrounding skin; an option is to apply a skin prepping solution to the area round the wound.

(1) If the wound has no or a small to moderate amount of exudate (Figure 4):
   (a) Cleanse;
   (b) Apply hydrocolloid dressing;

   (c) Change 3 times per week and PRN if loose or soiled (NB The dressing may not adhere well to the buttocks when incontinence is a problem).

Or:
   (a) Cleanse;
   (b) Apply a transparent dressing;
   (c) Change every 3 days and PRN if loose or soiled – frequency must be specific but may be individualized.

(2) If the wound is on the buttocks and has very superficial multiple open areas and the patient is incontinent of bladder and/or bowel:
   (a) Cleanse buttocks and surrounding area with a commercial cleanser and dry;
   (b) Apply a second generation barrier cream;
   (c) Recleanse and reapply cream every shift. It is not necessary to remove all the old barrier cream with each cleansing, merely remove urine/feces or soiling before reapplying.

Stage III and stage IV treatment protocol

Wound cleansing: flush the wound with normal saline or commercial wound cleanser, dry the surrounding skin. A skin prepping solution may be applied to the surrounding area and allowed to dry.

(1) If the wound is dry or there is a small amount of exudate:
   (a) Cleanse;
   (b) Apply protective ointment to the intact skin immediately around the wound;
   (c) Apply hydrogel impregnated gauze to all wound surfaces;
   (d) Cover with a gauze or bordered gauze as appropriate; secure with tape;
   (e) Change dressing once a day.

(2) If the wound is shallow and has moderate to heavy exudate:
   (a) Cleanse (as above);
   (b) Apply protective ointment to intact skin immediately around the wound;

(c) Apply a foam dressing – there should be an overlap of approximately half an inch to an inch onto intact skin;

(d) Secure with tape. A bordered foam will require no other secondary dressing or tape;

(e) Change 3 times per week depending on the amount of exudate and saturation of the foam.

(3) If the wound has a cavity and has moderate to heavy exudate:

(a) Cleanse (as above);

(b) Apply protective ointment to the intact skin immediately around the wound;

(c) Pack the cavity with alginate dressing (rope);

(d) Cover with gauze and secure with tape;

(e) Change daily or q.o.d. depending on amount of exudate and/or saturation of the secondary dressing.

If the wound is tunneling, occlusive dressings must be avoided and the tunneling packed loosely with half-inch gauze packing saturated with normal saline or hydrogel to fill the dead space. The wound should then be dressed as in options 1, 2, or 3.

Eschar

Eschar is a form of necrotic tissue, and removal of the devitalized tissue is considered necessary for wound healing; the wound will appear larger as the debridement progresses. When a wound involves necrotic tissue, staging cannot be confirmed until its base is visible. The Agency for Health Care Policy and Research (AHCPR) guidelines recommend that heel ulcers with dry eschar need not be debrided if they do not have edema, erythema, fluctuance, or drainage. These wounds should be assessed daily to monitor for pressure ulcer complications that would require debridement (e.g. edema, erythema, fluctuance, drainage).

Treatment protocols

Surgical debridement is recommended for hard eschar, and the following protocol is designed to debride if surgical debridement is not done:

(1) Scrub the surface of the eschar tissue vigorously with normal saline using moist gauze at each dressing change;

(2) Cover the eschar with a transparent dressing;

(3) Change every 3 to 5 days. Frequency must be specific but individualized;

(4) Re-evaluate for new dressing option when the eschar has softened[11].

References

1. Norman RA. A dermatologist's guide to nursing home consultations. *J Geriatr Dermatol* 1998;6:62–77
2. Norman RA. How to manage wounds in long-term care patients. *J Geriatr Dermatol* 1999;7:50–6
3. Norman RA. Ten common dermatologic problems in the chronic care setting. *J Geriatr Dermatol* 2000;8:75–80
4. Norman RA, *et al*. Handling chronic and acute wounds in aging skin (panel discussion). *J Geriatr Dermatol* 1999;7:65–9
5. Coon WW, Willis PW, Keller JB. Venous thromboembolism and other venous disease in the Tecumseh Community Health Study. *Circulation* 1973;48:839–46
6. Rivlin AM, Wiener JM, Manley R, *et al*. Caring for the disabled elderly: who will pay? Washington, DC: The Brookings Institution, 1988:30–50
7. Panel for the prediction and prevention of pressure ulcers in adults. *Pressure Ulcers in Adults: Prediction and Prevention*. Clinical practice guideline number 3, AHCPR publication number 92-0047. Rockville, MD: Agency for Health Care Policy and Research, Public Health Service, US Department of Health and Human Services, May 1992

8. Sullivan DH. Impact of nutritional status on health outcomes of nursing home residents. *J Am Geriatr Soc* 1995;43:195
9. Young ME. Malnutrition and would healing. *Heart Lungs* 1988;17:60–7
10. Bergstrom N, *et al.* (Treatment of Pressure Ulcers Guideline Panel). Clinical Practice Guideline Number 15, US Department of Health and Human Services Public Health Service, Agency for Health Care Policy and Research, Rockville, Maryland: December 1994
11. Krasner D, ed. *Chronic Wound Care – A Clinical Source Book For Healthcare Professionals.* Health Management Publications, Inc., 1990

APPENDIX 1

Nursing-home dermatology consultation protocol

In this litigious age it is vital to ensure that the consultation is properly organized and co-ordinated with the director of nursing (or equivalent) and primary care doctor.

A skin condition check list (appendix 2), which is filled in by the duty nurse, can be useful in saving time while a skin care assessment (appendix 3) can be used to determine those who are at most risk and to monitor the course of treatment; incidentally, nursing-home visitations are often much more efficient than hospital ones. It might also be worthwhile having a standardized 'physician's order form' on hand (see appendix 4 for a sample).

Many nursing-home patients are just as mobile and clear-headed as are private-office patients and are able to give full consent if procedures are needed. If a patient is unable to give such consent, it is essential that the family or guardian be notified and the consent form signed before carrying out any procedures.

It is important to remember that one is visiting the patient's home when doing a consultation and to behave appropriately; it is essential that a male consultant be accompanied by a female aide or nurse when examining a female patient.

If the consultant is unable to take their own nursing assistant on a nursing-home visit the nursing director or floor supervisor will generally be able to provide someone who can assist with a surgery.

Inevitably it is impossible to have all the luxuries of the office at one's disposal in the nursing home, but the following are recommended: needles, xylocaine, shave biopsy tools, curettes, biopsy bottles and labels, scissors, scalpel, hemostat, pickups, suture, mini-cautery, a small cryotherapy container, a biological marker for excisions, Monsel's solution, alcohol pads, gauze, antibiotic ointment, tape and a biohazard bag for biological waste. A sharps container is also worth having available.

If 'physician extenders' – such as nurse practitioners and physician assistants – are employed, frequent follow-ups and chart reviews are recommended to make sure that the correct measures are being utilized in patient care. A good idea, especially at the beginning of the NP's or PA's career, is to have them take photographs – with consent – which can be brought back to the office for discussion of the patient's care.

Respect for the resident and his/her environment must be maintained. The entire group of employees and caretakers, including the attending physician, act as a surrogate family for the residents. A caring attitude and behavior make all the difference between one home and another, between a pleasant and rewarding experience and a degrading one.

APPENDIX 2

Sample: skin condition checklist

Date:....................   Name:....................   Room/Floor:....................

Nurse should investigate any areas of concern and write findings down on form for .... (dermatologist) or associate. Keep a list of all residents requiring skin consultation and notify the office when you have a group of residents to be seen.

Mark picture with the number please:

1. Open areas
2. Decubitus
3. Skin tear
4. Rashes
5. Bruise/Contusion
6. Swelling
7. Irregular texture/Tone-flaking, Scalp and/or Facial crusting, Inflammation/Reddened area, Pustules, Growths
8. Other

Comments...
....
....

*Put any applicable number(s) on area of body noted (example – if rash on left calf, put #4 on left calf)

....
Nurse's signature

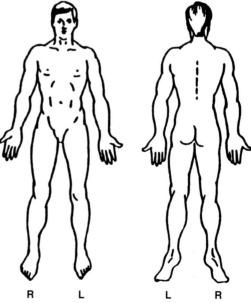

APPENDIX 3

Skin care assessment

Identify patient at risk of developing pressure ulcers by assessing and scoring.

*Braden scale (modified)

12 or < – high risk
13 or 14 – moderate risk
15 or 16 – low risk
16 or > – at risk

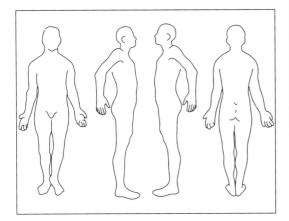

Draw a sketch of any impairment of skin integrity on the anatomical figures, number each sketch and describe below.

Description

#—— ————————————

#—— ————————————

#—— ————————————

#—— ————————————

Developed by: Barbara Braden and Nancy Bergstrom 1988

Feature assessed	Points
Sensory perception	
(Ability to respond to pressure)	
Completely limited	1
(Unresponsive)	
Very limited	2
(Responds to painful stimuli)	
Slightly limited	3
(Responds to verbal commands)	
No impairment	4
Moisture	
(Exposure to urine, perspiration, etc.)	
Constantly moist	1
(Detected every time moved)	
Very moist	2
(Linen/diaper/pad changed q. shift)	
Occasionally moist	3
(Extra change q. day)	
Rarely moist	4
Activity	
(Degree of physical activity)	
Bedfast	1
(Confined to bed)	
Chairfast	2
(Non weight-bearing)	
Walks occasionally	3
(Short distance walks)	
No limitations	4
Mobility	
(Ability to change and control body position)	
Completely immobile	1
(Requires assistance to move)	
Very limited	2
(Infrequent changes)	
Slightly limited	3
(Frequent/slight changes)	
No limitations	4
Nutrition	
(Usual food intake)	
Very poor	1
(Never completes meal/npo IVs or liquids > 5 days)	
Probably inadequate	2
(< 3 servings protein, ½ meal)	
Adequate	3
(> ½ meal, 4 servings protein)	
Excellent	4
Friction/shear	
Problem	1
(Constant friction)	
Potential problem	2
(Moves feebly/some sliding)	
No apparent problem	3
(Maintains good position)	
	Score

APPENDIX 4

Sample physician's order form

Wound care orders   Date:......................

1. Complete blood count, SMA-25, transferrin, and serum zinc level

2. Repeat SMA-25 and CBC every two weeks; please co-ordinate with other necessary blood tests if possible

3. Use protective measures on all wounds, including mattress overlay, heel and elbow protectors, and pillows and foam wedges on ankles, knees and other pressure sites

4. Keep weight off wound sites at all times

5. Reposition resident at least every two hours

6. Physical therapy to screen and evaluate wounds with weekly follow-up

7. Dietician to evaluate and follow patient

8. Multi-vitamin – one tablet per day

9. Vitamin C 500 mg p.o. t.i.d.

10. Folic Acid 1 mg p.o. daily

11. Zinc sulphate tabs 220 mg p.o. q. a.m. for 10 days if serum zinc level below 600–1200 mcg/l

12. Orange juice 3 oz with each meal

13. Psychiatric or psychological consult if patient depressed

14. If wound is on leg, obtain arterial ultrasound of both legs

15. House supplement t.i.d.

16. Give all medications by feeding tube if necessary, or may crush or use liquid alternative

17. Review care plan every week and update as necessary

18. Refer resident to wound/skin care committee if available

19. Monitor granulation of wound bed weekly and document site and stage of wound and granulation

20. Do not use iodine compounds or hydrogen peroxide in any form relating to wound treatment

21. If wound gets worse or does not respond as expected, please call my office

22. Please notify family/responsible party of wound care protocol and progress, or lack of, towards healing of wound

Physician's signature:...

Patient's name:......................................   Room number:...

Skin diseases of the elderly

S. L. Moschella

INTRODUCTION

In both developed and underdeveloped countries the proportion of the elderly is increasing, and in the twenty-first century the number of older people will double or even triple[1].

The two basic theories of aging are the programmatic theory which postulates aging genes, cellular senescence, telemere shortening and failure of apoptosis and longevity genes, and the stochastic theory of oxidative stress, amino acid racemization, and nonenzymatic glycosylation. There is also the possibility of decremental failure of the immune system. Skin change is affected by two phenomena: true aging due to the passage of time, and photoaging resulting from exposure to the sun[2].

The functions of the skin that decline with age are cell replacement, barrier function, chemical clearance, sensory perception, mechanical protection, wound healing, immune responsiveness, thermoregulation, sweat and sebum production, vitamin D production and DNA repair[3].

The cutaneous signs of aging in skin that has not been exposed to light are xerosis (dryness), fine wrinkling, thinning of skin and loss of elasticity and the development of seborrheic keratoses and skin tags[4]. In the elderly, skin that has been exposed to the sun is hypopigmented and mottled with blotchy erythema and has coarse deep wrinkling and an increased incidence of epidermal dysplasia and malignant lesions. Table 1 is a list of dermatologic disorders[5].

Senile pruritus or xerosis

One of the most frequent and disturbing eruptions in the elderly is generalized itching. It is

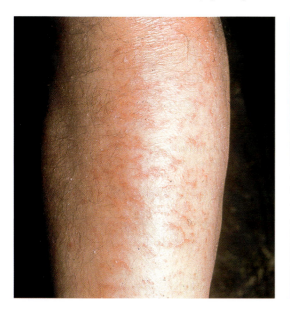

Figure 1 Asteatotic eczema (eczema craquelé)

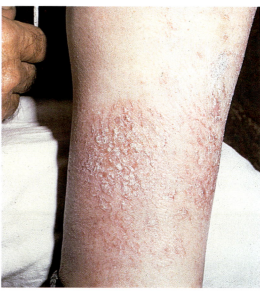

Figure 2 Xerosis with eczematization

Table 1   Dermatologic disorders

Senile pruritus	*Neoplasia*
	Benign
Eczematous dermatitis	Cherry angiomas, skin tags, colloid milium,
Asteatotic eczema	cutaneous horns, seborrheic keratosis, sebaceous
Nummular eczema	hyperplasia, clear cell acanthoma, keratoacanthoma
Seborrheic dermatitis	*Malignant*
Gravitational eczema	Basal cell cancer, Bowen's disease, squamous cell
Autoeczematization eczema	cancer, lentigo maligna melanoma, Kaposi's
Psychogenic dermatitides (lichen simplex, prurigo	sarcoma, angiosarcoma, cutaneous T and B cell
nodularis and neurotic excoriations, delusions	lymphoma, leukemia cutis
of parasitosis)	
Ulcers complicating diabetic insensitivity	*Erythroderma*
	Psoriasis
Infections	Pityriasis rubra pilaris
Bacterial	Sezary's syndrome
Dermatophyte	Drug
Candidiasis	
Pyoderma, folliculitis, cellulitis	*Paraneoplastic syndrome*
Herpes zoster	Erythema gyratum repens
	Hypertrichosis lanuginosa acquisita
Infestations	Subcutaneous fat necrosis of adults
Scabies	Sweet's syndrome
Pediculosis	Acrokeratosis paraneoplastic (Bazex's syndrome)
	Acanthosis nigricans
Transient acantholytic disease (Grover's disease)	Acquired keratoderma of the palms and soles
	Paraneoplastic pemphigus and pemphigus vulgaris
Disorders of nutrition	Necrolytic migratory erythema
Zinc deficiency	Multicentric reticulohistiocytosis
Scurvy	Vasculitis
Pellagra	Dermatomyositis
	Pachydermoperiostosis
Autoimmune disorders	
Blistering	*Disorders of the mucous membranes*
Bullous pemphigoid	Cheilitis
Pemphigus vulgaris	Perlèche
Cicatrizing pemphigoid	Leukoplakia
Epidermolysis bullosa acquisita	Oral cancer
Immune rheumatologic disorders	
Sjogren's disease	*Disorders of the ano-genital area*
Dermatomyositis	Pruritus ani, vulvae
Small vessel vasculitis	Atrophic vulvitis
Giant cell arteritis	Lichen sclerosis et atrophicans
Wegner's granulomatosis	Balanitis xerotica obliterans
Amyloidosis	Squamous cell cancer of the penis and vulva
Vascular disorders	*Disorders of the feet*
Chilblains	Clavi, corns, calluses
Erythema ab igne	Subungual exostosis
Lichen aureus	Dystrophic nail changes
Chronic venous insufficiency and varicose ulcer	
Atheroembolism, ischemia and gangrene	*Disorders of the hair*
	Androgenic alopecia
Photosensitivity disorders	Graying
Actinic reticuloid	Senescence alopecia
Phototoxic and photoallergic drug reactions	

usually unassociated with any dermatologic or systemic disease. The skin is dry, rough, scaly and consistent with asteatosis (Figure 1). The pruritus usually is worse during the winter and is aggravated by frequent bathing especially with hot water and 'strong' detergents. When the patient takes his or her clothes off in the evening, they may experience intense fits of pruritus. Low humidity and temperatures during winter months are contributory. The itching can lead to excoriations, which can be secondarily eczematized and infected with staphylococci. The conditions to be ruled out are irritant or contact dermatitis from topical medications and preparations and the occasional association with an underlying lymphoproliferative disease (lymphoma or leukemia) or systemic disease (diabetes and hepatic and renal disorder), or drugs.

Eczematous dermatitis

Eczematous dermatitis is one of the most frequent dermatologic problems[6]. It can be complicating asteatosis (Figure 2), nummular eczema (Figure 3), acute contact irritant dermatitis (Figure 4), infectious eczematoid dermatitis (Figure 5), stasis eczema and a psychogenic dermatosis induced by rubbing or mechanical friction. Nummular eczema consists of extremely pruritic well-marginated, vesiculated 'weeping' plaques which crust and develop scales (Figure 3). It can be acute or subacute. The eruption can be widespread but favors the extremities. The skin tends to be dry and not infrequently associated with atopy. Because of the discoid nature of the lesions the condition must be differentiated from psoriasis and tinea corporis.

Seborrheic dermatitis is characterized by flaking of the scalp and dry, red, scaly skin of the face, trunk and anogenital region (Figure 6). The increased incidence and severity seen in patients with Parkinson's disease, quadriplegia and emotional distress suggests that the condition is influenced by the central nervous system. The condition can be effectively treated by use of an antifungal shampoo and application of a mild steroid cream.

Stasis dermatitis (Figure 7) usually occurs with venous insufficiency, varicose veins, and pedal edema. It results from venous hypertension and deep vein thrombosis. There is a brownish discoloration of the skin from hemosiderin deposition. Chronic eczematous dermatitis occurs around the ankles (Figure 7a). Trauma can cause ulceration (Figure 7b). Among the complications of the dermatitis and/or ulcer are cellulitis and contact dermatitis from topical medications, especially antibiotics. Some topical medications or a complicating infection can induce autosensitization – the so-called 'Id' reaction – which can produce a symmetrical eczematous dermatitis especially of the extremities and/or a dyshidrotic eczematous dermatitis of the hands and feet.

The elderly, because of disease and socioeconomic conditions, are often subject to stress and experience anxiety and/or depression as a result of which psychogenic disorders can be seen. Lichen simplex chronicus usually affects individuals with an obsessive personality who focus on pruritic lesions. These patients usually have an atopic background and are prone to scratch their skin or rub an antecedent dermatitis. Diffuse lichenification can result in the so-called leonine facies (Figure 8). The lesions can be single or multiple but are always within the reach of the fingers. The common sites of involvement are the nape of the neck (so-called 'nuchal dermatitis'), extensor surface of the elbows, flexor surfaces of wrists and ankles, the anogenital region, the external auditory meatus and the palms and soles. The lesions are poorly marginated, lichenified, scaling erythematous plaques, which must be differentiated sometimes from psoriasis, a fungal infection or mycosis fungoides. The anogenital pruritus may have significant psychosexual overtones but can be triggered by fecal contamination. Conditions to be ruled out are vaginal infections, pinworm parasitization, diabetes mellitus, lichen sclerosis et atrophicans and psoriasis.

Prurigo nodularis may present as an abnormality of the sensory nerve innervation of the skin. It is characterized by scattered discrete keratotic pigmented nodules on the extremities, especially in middle-aged women. The itching is very intense and even painful. Three conditions to be considered in the differential

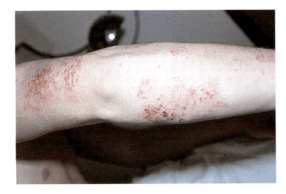

Figure 3   Nummular eczema in a patient with atopic eczema

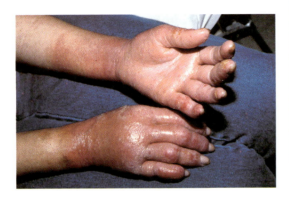

Figure 4   Acute contact dermatitis associated with the use of cleansing solution

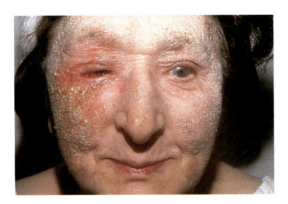

Figure 5   Patient with infectious conjunctivitis developed a periocular eczematous dermatitis about the eye which is described as an infectious eczematoid dermatitis

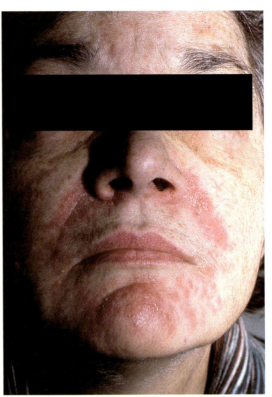

Figure 6   Seborrheic dermatitis of the face

diagnosis are hypertrophic lichen planus, cutaneous amyloidosis, actinic prurigo and bullous pemphigoid.

Neurotic excoriations are, to a certain extent, self-inflicted conditions, though they may be preceded by a causative factor such as an insect bite or rubbing. Patients compulsively pick their skin, and this gives rise to lesions in all stages of development including ulcerations, nodules and atrophic scars.

Diabetic patients can develop peripheral sensory neuropathy with complicating skin ulceration secondary to trauma or constant pressure (decubitus) (Figure 9).

Delusions of parasitosis are characterized by complaints about a crawling sensation which, the patient is convinced, is produced by parasites. Such patients – most of whom are female – support their belief by producing 'material' dug out of their skin. The attending physician is unable to find any parasite or its by-products on examination. Among the contributing factors are psychosis, psychoneurosis, toxic states, nutritional deficiencies, drug addiction and arteriosclerosis.

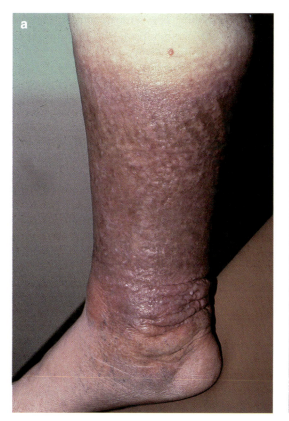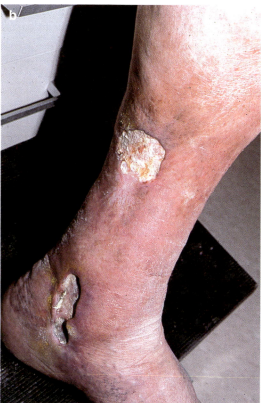

Figure 7   (a) Stasis dermatitis with underlying dermato-liposclerosis. (b) Stasis ulcers

Skin infections

Skin infections of the elderly can be bacterial, fungal or viral[6]. Among the bacterial infections are impetigo (streptococcal), characterized by pruritic honey-colored crusted erosions, bullous impetigo (staphylococcal), consisting of thin-walled flaccid bullae, and erysipelas (streptococcal cellulitis) which manifests as well defined plaques especially on the face, scalp and perineum and is often misdiagnosed as psoriasis.

The fungal infections are dermatophytosis and candidiasis. The dermatophyte involvement is mainly tinea pedis, onychomycosis and tinea cruris. Tinea pedis is usually an erythematous scaling dermatitis with a moccasin-like presentation (Figure 10), with or without interdigital and dystrophic nail changes. Tinea cruris is a pruritic circinate erythematous scaling eruption of the groin. Tinea unguium is clinically a dull opaque yellowish-white discoloration of the nails, which can become brittle, friable, hypertrophic and dystrophic. The diagnosis in all these clinical expressions is confirmed by demonstration of the septate branching hyphae under the microscope or a specific type of growth on Sabaroud's culture medium. Candidal infection favors intertriginous moist areas i.e. flexural, submammary, . anogenital and perioral (Figure 11). The eruption usually consists of 'beef-red' weeping areas with satellite pustules; it sometimes presents as inflammatory arcuate lesions, usually in the groin. The paronychial area can be involved especially in those who are diabetic and/or have their hands repeatedly wet. Again, the diagnosis is confirmed by demonstration of pseudohyphae and spores on microscopy or its characteristic growth on culture. The predisposing conditions are diabetes, antibiotics, nutritional factors and diminished salivary function.

Two viral infections may affect the aged. Herpes zoster is seen most frequently in the aged, especially in individuals immuno-suppressed by disease or therapy. The patient usually complains of pain, tenderness and hyperesthesia of the dermatome that later develops painful clusters of small umbilicated vesicles. The pain (post zoster neuralgia) may last for weeks, months, or years. About 5% of patients may develop a varicelliform erup-tion outside the involved dermatome. Complicating motor changes can involve the urinary bladder, rectal sphincter and bowel. Involvement of the ophthalmic branch of the facial nerve can cause corneal ulceration. Molluscum contagiosum, a type of poxvirus, although most commonly seen in children also occurs in the elderly. The lesion consists of pinkish-white dome-shaped and umbili-cated papules. One the face, especially if it is solitary, it can be misdiagnosed as a basal cell cancer.

Parasitic infestations

Two parasitic infestations occur in the elderly, scabies and pediculosis[7]. Although scabies in the aged may present in an atypical fashion, it usually presents in the classical clinical expression as small extremely pruritic excori-ated papules of fingers, wrists, elbows, ante-rior axillary field, breasts, genitals, buttocks and abdomen (Figure 12). However, in the elderly there is usually less inflammation but the pruritus is still intense and the back, an unusual site, maybe involved. In institutions or hospitals the aged may acquire Norwegian scabies, which clinically presents as a crusted exfoliative erythroderma with involvement of the nails, palms and soles. The lesion contains myriads of mites. The diagnosis is made by demonstration in skin scrapings of any stage of the mite, eggs and typical fecal pellets. The lice infestations are pediculosis capitis (head lice), pediculosis corporis (vagabond's disease, body lice), and pediculosis pubis (crab lice,

pubic lice). The lice and/or nits should be looked for in the scalp, axilla, or pubic hair and in clothing seams. Pediculosis pubis causes a pruritic eruption with demonstrable nits in the hair and the adult organisms in the pubis. In the aged the eyelashes can be involved.

Grover's disease

Transient acantholytic dermatosis[7] (Grover's disease) (Figure 13) is common in men over 40 years of age; its cause is unknown. It can be persistent. Clinically there are scattered pru-ritic erythematous papules or papulovesicles with crusting on the neck, upper chest, back and trunk. Histologically there are acantholy-sis and dyskeratosis.

Nutritional disorders

The elderly may suffer secondary vitamin defi-ciencies from inappropriate diet or from underlying diseases[7]. Scurvy and pellagra are examples. Clinically scurvy is characterized by perifollicular hyperkeratotic papules with centrally curved hairs surrounded by ery-thema and purpura. Hemorrhage can occur in the skin as ecchymosis, in the gingiva, gastrointestinal tract, central nervous system, the genitourinary tract and subperiosteum. Pellagra results from deficiency of tryptophan and/or of vitamins of the B complex, especially nicotinic acid. The clinical manifestations are due to photosensitivity and are erythema, edema with vesiculation, and blistering. As the acute eruption subsides, the skin becomes rough, fissured and blackish-brown.

Autoimmune disorders

Among autoimmune blistering disorders not infrequently seen in the aged are bullous pemphigoid, cicatrizing pemphigoid and pemphigus vulgaris. Bullous pemphigoid (Figure 14) usually occurs in the elderly and is more frequent in women. It is the most common autoimmune disorder in the Western world. Among the drugs that have been associated with bullous pemphigoid

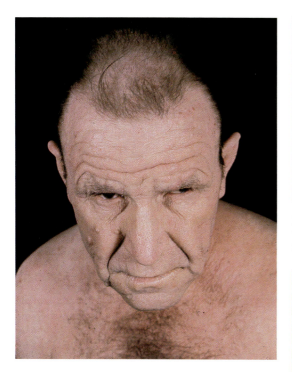

Figure 8 Chronic resistant atopic eczema in a patient with chronic asthma

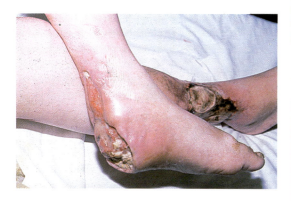

Figure 9 Patient has diabetes mellitus with peripheral neuropathy and insensitivity with complicating ulcerations

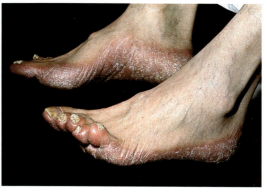

Figure 10 Chronic fungus infection (Tinea rubrum) of the skin and nails of 15 years' duration with a 'moccasin' like clinical presentation

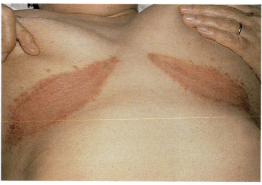

Figure 11 Submammary intertriginous candidiasis in a diabetic patient

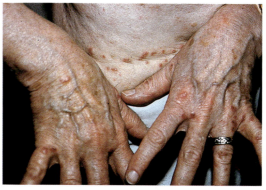

Figure 12 Excoriated papulovesicular lesions between fingers and on abdomen, buttocks and scrotum resulting from scabetic infestation

are furosemide, sulfasalazine, penicillins, capitrol, antipsychotic drugs and aldosterone antagonists. An association with malignancy is controversial. The patient may present with pruritus for weeks or months before the onset of blistering. It can also present as an erythematous pruritic urticarial dermatitis or an eczematous process before the onset of blistering. A figurative erythema with marginal vesiculation may be another clinical expression. Non-inflamed bullae may present on the lower extremities as the so-called bullous

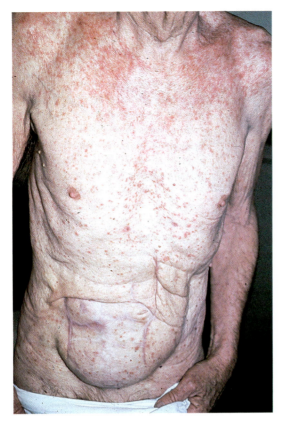

Figure 13   Patient with pruritic papulovesicular eruption of the chest and abdomen consistent with transient acantholytic disease

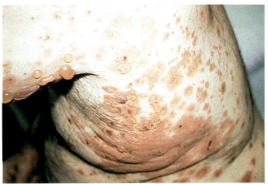

Figure 14   Bullous pemphigoid exhibiting erythematous plaques with blistering

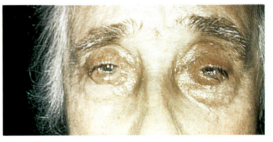

Figure 15   Cicatrizing pemphigoid with resulting conjunctival scarring and resulting blindness

eruption of the aged. The lesions usually appear as, tense pruritic bullae on erythematous or normal appearing skin favoring the flexural areas of the extremities and lower abdomen. Mucosal blistering is rare but a desquamative gingivitis may occur. It is a subepidermal blistering disease. The presence of the third component of complement C3 and IgG at the basement membrane are the immunopathologic findings.

Cicatrizing pemphigoid (Figure 15) is a subepithelial blistering disorder involving skin and mucous membranes and results in scarring in these areas. The lesions involve the oral conjunctiva and the nasopharyngeal, laryngeal, esophageal, genital and rectal mucosa. Skin lesions occur in one third of cases and favor the scalp, face and upper trunk. They appear as tense bullae and erosions. The disease tends to be chronic and progressive. On direct immunofluorescence there are immunoreactants (mainly IgG and C3 but also IgA and IgM) in the epithelial basement membranes. A localized form of this disease, the so-called Brunsting–Perry pemphigoid, is characterized by recurrent localized subepidermal blistering and scarring of the head and neck.

Pemphigus vulgaris is a non-scarring, blistering disorder of the skin and mucous membranes, characterized by flaccid blisters on erythematous skin which easily ruptures and leaves denuded areas. Mucous membranes, especially the mouth, are frequently involved. Pemphigus usually affects middle-aged people of all races and both sexes, although there is an increased susceptibility in Jewish people, especially Ashkenazi Jews. Patients appear to be genetically predisposed to other autoimmune

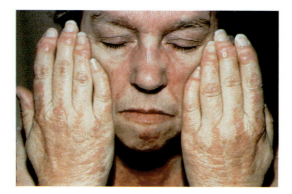

Figure 16 Dermatomyositis in patient with carcinoma of the breast

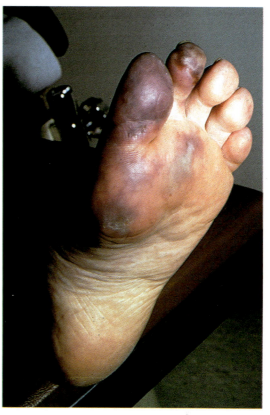

Figure 17 Patient who has a severe arteriosclerosis with a history of stroke, is on warfarin and developed atheroembolism

diseases. Clinically it may present as a localized disease, especially in the mouth, scalp or nose, months before the skin is involved. The skin areas of predilection are scalp, face, axillae, groin and flexural sites. Lesions on the scalp and flexural areas may become vegetative (pemphigus vegetans). Nail involvement can cause dystrophy and paronychia. Histopathology of skin lesions reveals supra-basal cell clefting with acantholytic cells in a blister cavity. The immunopathology reveals IgG autoantibodies, which bind demoglein 3 (target antigen) in the desmosomes and the cell membrane of keratinocytes.

Pemphigus foliaceus (superficial pemphigus) is seen less frequently than pemphigus vulgaris. In rural areas of South America an endemic form of the disease is seen. The eruption usually involves the seborrheic areas such as the scalp, face, chest and back, and presents clinically as crusted erosions which are painful and have an offensive odor. Sometimes patients present with or develop an exfoliative erythroderma. Histopathology, superficial clefts and bullae are seen immediately below the stratum corneum or high in the granular layer. The bullae contain scattered granular acantholytic keratinocytes, neutrophils and fibrin. Eosinophilic or neutrophilic spongiosis can precede the above changes. The autoantibodies (IgG) recognize the target antigen demoglein 1, a 160-kDa desmosome cadherin.

Collagen vascular diseases[7] may have their onset in the aged but there is, in general, no greater incidence in the elderly and their clinical presentation is not unlike those seen more frequently in younger patients. Since malignancy is seen more often in the aged, dermatomyositis associated with malignancies are not infrequent. These patients can also have a cutaneous eruption like dermatomyositis (Figure 16) without demonstrable myositis (dermatomyositis sine myositis).

Sjögrens syndrome is an autoimmune disorder characterized by dryness of mucus membranes of the eyes, mouth and vagina. It may be associated with rheumatoid arthritis. Biopsy of lip demonstrating lymphohistocystic infiltrate in minor salivary gland is diagnostic.

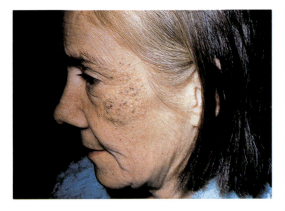

Figure 18 Nodular elastosis with comedone formation (Favre–Rachouchot syndrome)

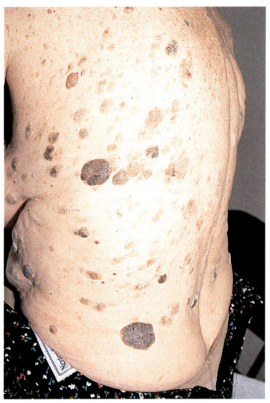

Figure 20 Disseminated seborrheic keratoses

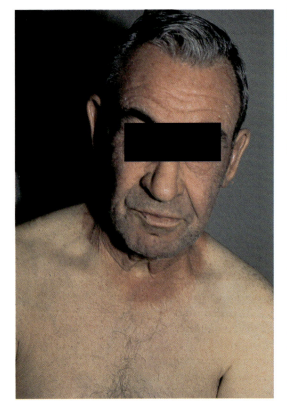

Figure 19 Actinic reticulated dermatitis precipitated by the fragrance in an after-shave lotion

Vascular disorders

Chronic vascular insufficiency is caused by venous hypertension secondary to valvular incompetence, and can be exacerbated by prolonged standing and venous thrombosis; there may also be hereditary factors involved. It may manifest as edema, varicosities, brown discoloration, superficial neovascularization, dermatitis and venous ulcers (most commonly on the medial lower leg – see chapter 10).

Cutaneous cholesterol embolism appears in patients with severe arteriosclerosis (Figure 17). The atheroembolism results from cholesterol crystals, which become detached from atheromatous plaques; it may occur spontaneously or complicate intravascular studies and surgical procedures. The microemboli affect small arteries and arterioles of the viscera – gastrointestinal tract, kidney – and the central nervous system and retina. The cutaneous manifestations are paroxysmal painful ischemia of the feet and legs, livedo reticularis, gangrene (i.e. 'warfarin' toes) and ulcers. The differential diagnosis includes the coagulopathy syndromes and periarteritis nodosa.

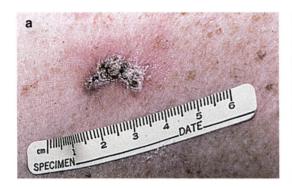

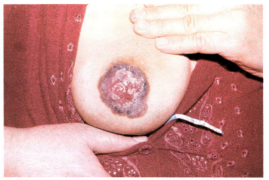

Figure 22   A 'weeping' plaque lesion of the breast of 3 years' duration; Paget's disease

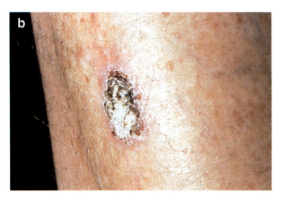

Figure 21   (a) Three tender actinic keratoses of the chest. (b) Hypertrophic actinic keratoses of the leg

Photosensitivity disorders

The sun in the aged causes photoaging or dermatoheliosis, cutis rhomboidalis nuchae, solar lentigo, Favre–Rachouchot syndrome (Figure 18), senile purpura, venous lake and stellate scars of the upper extremities. One of the hypersensitivity reactions seen in the elderly is actinic reticuloid dermatitis. In fair-skinned elderly photoaging is characterized by roughness and atrophy of the skin, loss of fat, wrinkling and pigmentary changes on areas exposed to light. In chronically photodamaged skin solar elastotic syndrome (characterized by an accumulation of elastotic material in the dermis), cutis rhomboidalis nuchae (characterized by coarse furrows in the thickened, leathery skin of the neck) and Favre–Rachouchot syndrome (Figure 18) (consisting of nodular elastosis with cysts and comedones) are frequently observed. Among the pigmented lesions created by chronic exposure to sunlight are senile lentigo with

pigmented macules in light exposed areas, especially the face and the dorsa of the hands, and reticulated pigmented and erythematous eruption of the neck (poikiloderma-like) sparing the submental area. The vascular changes are solar purpura secondary to trauma in light-exposed areas, venous ectasia (i.e. venous lake) on the lower lip, often misdiagnosed as melanoma or pigmented basal carcinoma, and the tearing of the fragile skin creating purpura and stellate scarring of the dorsum of the hands and forearms.

Actinic reticuloid dermatitis is a photosensitivity disorder associated with exaggerated response to UVA or UVB and even visible light. Some patients have a history of contact allergy to oleoresin extracts of common fragrances and composite plants. Clinically, the patients have lichenified erythematosus plaques of the forehead and neck which can progress to create a leonine facies (Figure 19). The itching is very intense. It has been described as a pseudolymphoma, but there are reports of a transition to malignant lymphoma. The histopathologic infiltrate is predominately T-cell suppressor cells (OKT_8).

Since older people are often on multiple drugs, photosensitivity drug reactions are apt to occur. Among the drugs responsible are thiazide diuretics and sulfonamide-based hypoglycemic agents. Patients on naproxen and furosemide may develop porphyria-like eruptions on areas of skin that have been exposed to the sun.

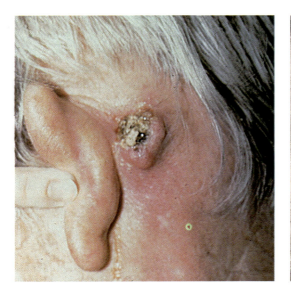

Figure 23   Keratoacanthoma of the retroauricular area; duration of 4 months

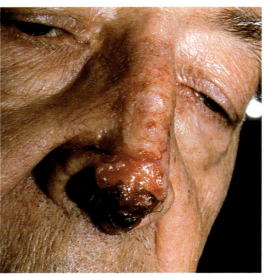

Figure 24   Recurrent basal cell cancer after inadequate excision

Neoplasia

The tumors seen are benign cherry angiomas, seborrheic keratosis, actinic keratosis and leukoplakia. Among the intraepidermal neoplasias are Bowen's disease (squamous cell cancer *in situ*), extramammary Paget's disease (adenocarcinoma *in situ*) and lentigo maligna disease. Among the epidermal carcinomas are keratoacanthoma, basal cell cancer, squamous cell carcinoma and melanoma. Among the dermal neoplasms are microcystic adnexal carcinoma, angiosarcoma, Kaposi's sarcoma, atypical fibroxanthoma, Merkel cell cancer and T cell lymphomas[8].

Cherry angiomas are multiple bright red to purplish, smooth 1–3 mm papules on the trunk and proximal extremities. Seborrheic keratoses (Figure 20) are the most common tumor, and occur symmetrically on the face, back, chest, abdomen and proximal extremities. These benign lesions are tan to dark brown or black flat or domed verrucous papules and appear to be stuck on the skin. Actinic keratosis (solar or senile keratosis) (Figure 21a&b) is a red to brown rough keratotic papule, measuring 3–6 mm in diameter, on sun damaged skin. Leukoplakia is seen in the elderly, especially smokers and tobacco chewers, and presents as whitish patches on the mucosal surface, often with epithelial dysplasia and with about 10% developing squamous cell carcinoma.

Bowen's disease, an intraepithelial squamous cell carcinoma which usually appears on exposed areas and on the mucous membranes, is called erythroplasia of Queyrat. Bowen's disease favors fair-complexioned men. Sunlight and arsenic ingestion are believed to be causative. About 30% have multiple lesions. In 5% of patients it evolves into invasive squamous carcinoma. Paget's disease and extramammary Paget's disease are other intraepithelial carcinomas. The breast lesion (Paget's disease) is associated with underlying ductal carcinoma of the breast (Figure 22). Extramammary Paget's disease most commonly affects the vulva and male genitalia, perianal area and the axillae. The lesion is a sharply marginated erythematous oozing plaque which may itch. Extramammary Paget's disease represents in some cases an extension of an underlying adenocarcinoma.

Keratoacanthoma (Figure 23) is a rapidly growing reddish papule with a central keratin plug; it is benign and spontaneously regresses. Histologically and clinically it resembles a

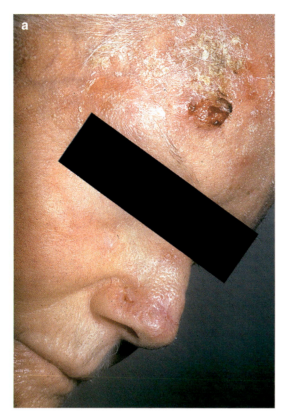
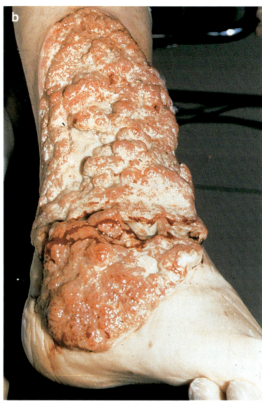

Figure 25 (a) Squamous cell carcinoma of the forehead. (b) Squamous cell carcinoma complicating a previous burn site

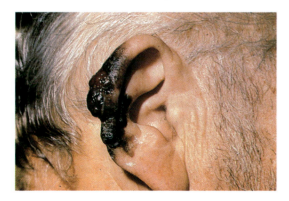

Figure 26 Lentigo maligna with melanoma. He had a flat pigmented lesion for 6 years and within the last year noted a more rapidly growing pigmented nodule in the lesion

well-differentiated squamous cell carcinoma and it appears most frequently in men on skin that has been exposed to the sun.

Basal cell carcinoma is the most common malignancy of humans (Figure 24). There are three types, nodular-ulcerative, sclerosing and superficial (multicentric). The most common type, the nodulo-ulcerative, favors the face and is a translucent erythematous papule, nodule or plaque with telangiectatic vessels. The sclerosing lesion is a yellowish-white sclerotic plaque and superficial basal cell carcinoma is an inflammatory lesion with an elevated thin border, usually multiple, and resembles psoriasis.

Squamous cell carcinoma (Figure 25a) favors fair-skinned individuals, is more common in men, occurs on areas that have been exposed to the sun and usually arises from an actinic keratosis or Bowen's disease. When actinic keratosis evolves into a squamous cell cancer, the original lesion becomes more inflamed and indurated. The *de novo* lesion rapidly enlarges and becomes ulcerated

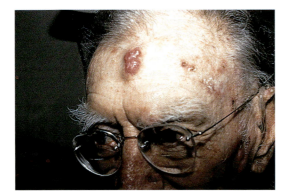

Figure 27   Merkel cell tumor, a slowly growing nodule of 1.5 years' duration

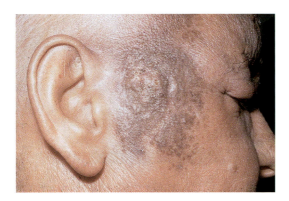

Figure 28   Angiosarcoma of the face of a 55-year-old male

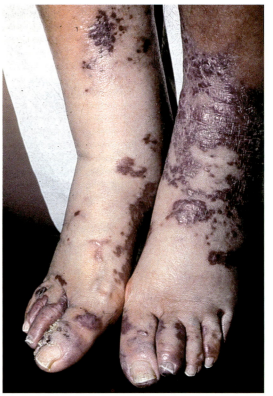

Figure 29   Hemorrhagic plaques of 15 years' duration, classic endemic Kaposi's sarcoma

centrally. Squamous cell cancers arising in sun-damaged skin have a low tendency to metastasize (0.5–3%). However, squamous cell cancer can arise in previously damaged tissue, for example burn scars (Figure 25b), and sinus tracts, and is more aggressive with a higher incidence of metastasis.

There has been an increase in the incidence of malignant melanoma especially in young Caucasian women. The lifetime risk in Caucasians is about one in eighty. The lesion may arise *de novo* or from pre-existing lesions such as a nevus or lentigo maligna. There are four primary types of malignant melanoma: superficial spreading, nodular, acrolentiginous and lentigo maligna. Its prognosis is proportional to the thickness of the tumor (Breslow thickness). Lentigo maligna melanoma comprises about 5% of melanoma. Lentigo maligna

melanoma (Figure 26) is a brown-black macule with irregular borders and uneven pigmentation. The lesion tends to be large in females and to occur mainly in middle-aged and older people. Areas exposed to the sun, especially the face, are the usual sites involved. It progresses to malignant melanoma after a period of 10–15 years in 30–50% of patients.

Microcystic adnexal carcinoma (MAE) is a locally aggressive cutaneous neoplasm found especially in women and has follicular and sweat gland differentiation. It involves the face, especially the upper lip and periorbital areas. It is neurotropic and rarely if ever metastasizes. Malignant fibrous histiocytoma is the most common soft tissue sarcoma of late adult life; it favors males appearing most commonly on the thighs and lower extremities. It is flesh-colored and is occasionally

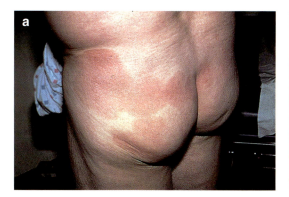

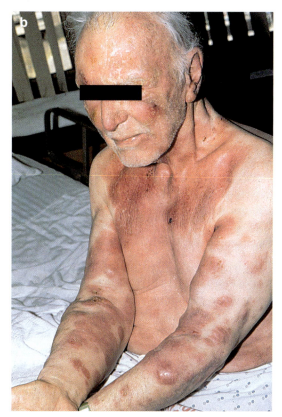

Figure 30 (a) Patch type of mycosis fungoides. (b) Plaque and nodules of mycosis fungoides

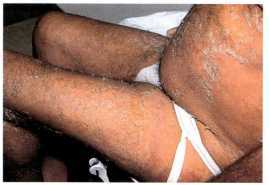

Figure 31 Exfoliative erythroderma in a patient with psoriasis of 20 years' duration

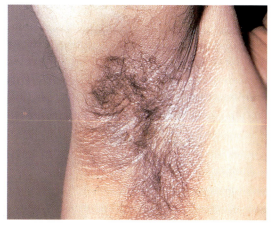

Figure 32 Acanthosis nigricans in patient with carcinoma of the stomach

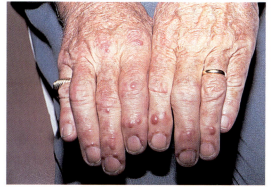

Figure 33 Classic distribution of erythematous firm non-tender nodules on fingers and paronychial area ('beading') in patient with multicentric reticulohistiocytosis and with prostatic cancer

ulcerated. It may complicate chronic ulcers, burn scars, surgical and irradiation sites. Metastasis occurs within 2 years. Atypical fibroxanthoma is a low-grade malignancy occurring in sun-exposed areas of the head and neck of the elderly. Because of its relatively small size and superficial origin it has a more favorable prognosis.

Merkel cell carcinoma (Figure 27) is a malignant neuroendocrine tumor with features of epithelial differentiation. It occurs in patients older than 65 years of age. It clinically presents as solitary, violaceous-red dome-shaped nodules with overlying telangiectasis and occurs most frequently on the head and neck. There is a high incidence of recurrence with potential lymphatic and hematogenous metastasis.

Cutaneous angiosarcoma (Figure 28) usually affects elderly males. It has been associated with irradiation, vinyl chloride, anabolic steroids, and insecticides. It presents clinically as ill-defined bluish plaques with or without nodulation and ulceration and less frequently as erythematous woody edema and scarring alopecia. The scalp is most frequently involved; other sites are the nose, ears and lips. The cervical nodes, lung and liver are preferred sites of metastasis. The prognosis and 5-year survival rate are poor.

Kaposi's sarcoma (multiple idiopathic hemorrhagic sarcoma) (Figure 29) is a multicentric neoplastic vascular proliferation of endothelial-lined channels with aggregates of spindle shaped cells which primarily affects skin, especially of the lower legs and hands, and mucous membranes. The classic form is endemic and affects the elderly, especially those of central Europe (Jews, Poles, Russians) and Italians. There is occasionally an association with other primary malignancies especially of lymphoreticular origin.

Cutaneous T cell lymphoma (CTCL) includes a constellation of diseases of malignant clonal T lymphocytes which present initially on the skin. Mycosis fungoides and Sézary syndrome are the most common and their malignant cells are mature post-thymic T cells, usually helper/inducer (CD$_4$) phenotypes. Mycosis fungoides (MF) (Figure 30) most often affects male adults in their 5th decade and has a predilection for African-Americans. The lesions classically progress slowly over a period of 5 to 10 years through the defined cutaneous phases: erythematous scaly patches that may be poikilodermic, plaques and tumors (nodular and ulcerated). As MF advances, the chances of extra-cutaneous involvement increase. The most common sites are the regional lymph nodes, the lungs, liver, spleen, gastrointestinal tract and brain.

Erythroderma

Sézary syndrome is the erythrodermic leukemia variant of CTCL. Other potentially erythrodermic entities such as drug eruptions, atopic dermatitis, psoriasis (Figure 31) and contact dermatitis may mimic this entity. Since the clinical picture is not pathognomonic, the diagnosis is made by a combination of clinical, histopathologic and immunologic studies (monoclonal antibodies and gene rearrangement studies). Peripheral blood exhibits a leukocytosis with more than 10% hyperconvoluted cerebriforme nuclei. The syndrome may develop *de novo* and may be complicated by mycosis fungoides. Clinically, Sézary syndrome is an erythrodermic pruritic scaling dermatitis accompanied by palmo-plantar keratoderma, alopecia, onychodystrophy, adenopathy and hepatosplenomegaly. The patients can develop a leonine facies.

Paraneoplastic syndromes

Paraneoplastic syndromes[8] are cancer-associated conditions, which are not a direct part of the malignancy or a result of metastasis but occur frequently enough to make their presence significant. These syndromes may antedate, parallel, or be independent of the associated malignancy. Such syndromes are presented in Table 2.

Erythema gyratum repens is usually a rapidly changing and progressing gyrate scaling erythema which has a 'wood grain' pattern. The course of this disorder correlates well with the course of the associated malignancy of the lung, breast, upper gastrointestinal tract, and urogenital tract.

Hypertrichosis lanuginosa acquisita, so-called 'malignant down', is extremely rare and characterized by the sudden appearance of profuse soft, non-medullarly, nonpigmented downy hair ('dogface'). It has been most frequently associated with advanced malignancy

Table 2 Paraneoplastic syndromes with commonly associated neoplasms

Syndrome	Neoplasm
Erythema gyratum repens	Lungs, uterus, breast, upper GI tract
Hypertrichosis lanuginosa acquisita	Lung and colon
Subcutaneous fat necrosis of adults	Pancreas
Sweet's syndrome	Acute myelogenous leukemia
Acrokeratosis paraneoplastic (Bazex's syndrome)	Squamous cell of upper aerodigestive tract
Acanthosis nigricans	Abdominal 'hollow' viscera
Acquired keratoderma of palm and soles	GI tract, lung, bladder
Paraneoplastic pemphigus	Lymphoproliferative neoplasms
Necrolytic migratory erythema	Glucagonoma
Multicentric reticulohistiocytosis	Breast, cervix, ovary, lung
Vasculitis	Leukemia, lymphoma
Migratory thrombophlebitis	Pancreas
Dermatomyositis	Lung, breast, ovaries
Pachydermoperiostosis	Lung

of the lung, colon, breast and genitourinary tract.

Pancreatic carcinomas can be associated with two syndromes: subcutaneous fat necrosis and necrolytic migratory erythema. Subcutaneous fat necrosis in adults is characterized by the presence of tender erythematous nodules of the pretibial areas. It is frequently associated with polyarthralgia, fever and eosinophilia. There is an increased level of serum lipase, amylase and trypsin. Necrolytic migratory erythema is the cutaneous manifestation of glucagonoma syndrome. The patients have weight loss, weakness, diabetes, elevated plasma glucagon and hypoaminoacidemia. The mucocutaneous lesions are stomatitis and glossitis, annular or arciform erosive crusted macules or papules involving the central part of the face, lower abdomen, perineum and distal extremities.

Acrodermatitis paraneoplastic (Bazex's syndrome) is an erythematous scaling psoriasiform dermatosis of the bridge of the nose, ears and extremities. It is only seen in patients with carcinoma of the upper respiratory tract, upper digestive tract, and metastatic lymph node involvement of the cervical or mediastinal region.

Two blistering disorders that have been associated with malignant neoplasms are pemphigus vulgaris and paraneoplastic pemphigus. Pemphigus vulgaris is a blistering mucocutaneous disorder characterized by intraepithelial blistering with classic histopathologic and immunologic changes. The associated malignancies are thymoma and lymphoma, as well as tumors of the ovary, thyroid, breast, uterus and stomach. The paraneoplastic syndrome is characterized by mucocutaneous and polymorphous skin lesions with clinical features of erythema multiforme, lichen planus and pemphigus vulgaris. Histologically there is an interphase dermatitis with acantholysis (Figure 32) and keratinocyte necrosis with characteristic direct and indirect immunofluorescence and immunoprecipitation patterns in serum. It is associated with lymphoreticular neoplasms including lymphoma, chronic lymphocytic leukemia and benign thymoma.

Multicentric reticulohistiocytosis (Figure 33) (lipoid dermatoarthritis) is associated in approximately 25% of patients with visceral malignancies of the breast, cervix, ovary and lung. It is characterized clinically as an erythematous papular and nodular eruption of the fingers, extremities and mucous membranes. There is usually polyarthritis with cystic changes of the bone. The histopathologic picture is diagnostic.

Vasculitis can be a paraneoplastic syndrome. The vasculitides may be of small or medium size vessels with or without a granulomatous component. They are most frequently associated with leukemia and lymphoma.

References

1. Winker MA, Glass RM. The aging global population. A call for papers. *J Am Med Assoc* 1996:1758
2. Masoro EJ. Aging. In Masoro EJ, ed. *Current Concepts in Aging*. Oxford: Oxford University Press, 1995:3
3. Yaar M, Gilchrest BA. Aging skin. In Freedberg IM, Eisen AZ, Wo HK, *et al.*, eds. *Dermatology in General Medicine*, 5th edn. New York, McGraw-Hill, 1999:1697–706
4. Borkan GA, Norris AH. Assessment of biological aging using a profile of physical parameters. *J Gerontol* 1980;35:177–84
5. Havlick NL, Fitzpatrick TB, Kligman AM, Kligman LA. Geriatric dermatology. In Freedberg IM, Eisen AZ, Wo HK, *et al.*, eds. *Dermatology in General Medicine*, 5th edn. New York, McGraw-Hill, 1999:1707–23
6. Orkin M, Maibach M, Dahl MV. *Dermatology, a Lange Medical Book*. Norwalk: Appleton and Lange, 1991
7. Young EM, Newcomer VD, Kligman AM. *Geriatric Dermatology*. Philadelphia: Lea Febiger, 1993
8. Politi Y, Oplur J, Bremmer S. Cutaneous neoplastic syndromes. *Acta Derm Venereol (Stockh)* 1993;73:161–70

Geriatric hair and scalp disorders   4

J. L. Roberts

INTRODUCTION

Some hair and scalp conditions are more or less confined to the geriatric population while others are part of a continuum and are also seen in the earlier stages of adulthood. One thing that is constant, however, is the societal and psychological significance of hair loss[1-3]. Hair loss can be as devastating in older individuals as it is in younger ones. Hair loss is frequently the most traumatic side-effect for cancer patients, many of who are in the geriatric population[3]. The wise and wonderful woman in Figure 1 lost her hair to chemotherapy for leukemia at age 92. She felt that the loss of her hair ranked with the major losses she had suffered, including loss of a spouse, death of a child and diminished health owing to cancer. Others have stated that hair loss symbolizes the loss of other physical attributes and strength with the passing years. Scalp hair can be a source of pride or pain at any age. In addition, many older woman find themselves embarrassed by the newly emerging coarse facial hairs that they may not have the visual acuity to address.

GRAY AND WHITE HAIR

Gray or white hair is one of the more obvious signs of aging. Age of onset and extent of graying are genetically controlled and graying may occur as early as adolescence or be delayed until very advanced age. Figure 2 shows a woman in her mid-sixties whose hair began to go gray in her second decade; she has virtually a total absence of pigmented hair. Figure 3 shows a 93-year-old woman with only a few strands of gray or unpigmented hair. In both cases, hair density is excellent.

The beard and moustache gray first. Graying of the scalp hair begins at the sideburns and temples, then spreads to the vertex and lastly to the occipital area. On the average Caucasian scalp the first gray hairs typically appear in the mid-thirties, and in Negroid individuals this occurs about ten years later. Onset in Japanese is midway between these two. By age 50 years, the average Caucasian has about 50% gray scalp hair[4,5]. 'Gray' hair is visually an admixture of pigmented and unpigmented hair. 'Unpigmented' hairs can be gray or white. What exactly is the nature of gray or white hair and what mechanism is responsible for the expression of this trait? The answers are not precisely known. However, it is known that gray and white hairs differ. Gray hairs sustain a progressive reduction in the numbers of melanocytes with reduced productivity of the melanosomes they contain. Melanocytes are absent in white hairs[6]. Tyrosinase activity and DOPA reaction is progressively diminished in gray hair and absent in white hair[7]. Pigmentation is lost abruptly in a given follicle and it is unusual to see gradual loss of pigment along a hair shaft, suggesting that the ability of a follicle to produce pigment is lost in one of the early phases of anagen.

The suggestion that an individual's hair can turn gray or white overnight probably results from the selective shedding of pigmented hairs in alopecia areata with residual unpigmented hairs, already present, being spared[5].

In rare instances, premature graying can be associated with systemic or local pathology. Amyloidosis may present as whitening of the hair and hair loss. Repigmentation has been reported with treatment of the underlying

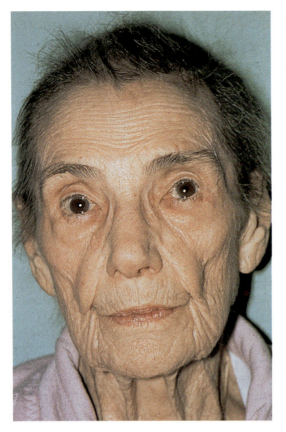

Figure 1 92-year-old woman with hair regrowth 4 months following chemotherapy for leukemia (anagen effluvium)

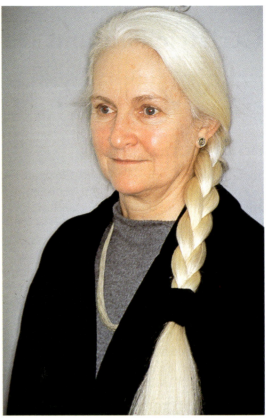

Figure 2 Woman in mid-sixties with totally white hair. Graying of hair began in teenage years

pathology[8]. It has been reported to occur with pernicious anemia[7], Addison's disease[9], hypothyroidism and, less commonly, with hyperthyroidism[9]. Locally, gray or white hair can be associated with regrowing hairs in alopecia areata. It appears to remain white more frequently in older individuals and may reflect an earlier expression of a genetic phenotype in these individuals. In addition, there is a higher incidence of concomitant autoimmune diseases in individuals with alopecia areata. Autoimmunity may be responsible for each of these organ-specific conditions and share a common mechanism[5]. The woman in Figure 4 developed late onset alopecia areata. She also had rheumatoid arthritis, type II diabetes, atopic dermatitis and vitiligo. Some authors have postulated that the inhibition or disappearance of melanogenesis in the normal graying process may be based on this principle.

Repigmentation has been reported to occur in the treatment of pernicious anemia[10], hypothyroidism, stabilized regrowth of alopecia areata, following electron beam therapy[11], erosive candidiasis of the scalp[12] and with large doses of para-aminobenzoic acid[13].

There have been two recent reports looking for any correlation between early graying and morbidity and mortality. In the prospective Copenhagen City Heart Study, which followed a random sample of 20 000 people over a 16-year period, no correlation was found between mortality and the extent of graying[14]. A second report of office and autopsy reports showed no correlation of early death or increased morbidity with early graying[15].

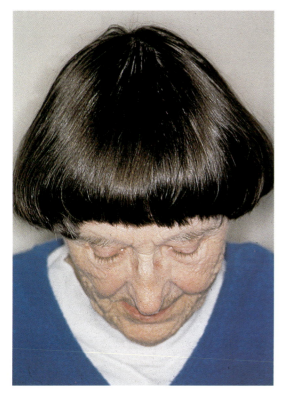

Figure 3   93-year-old woman with almost no graying of her hair

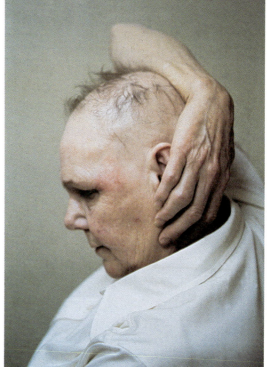

Figure 4   Woman with alopecia areata, vitiligo, rheumatoid arthritis and atopic dermatitis

HAIR GROWTH CHARACTERISTICS

There are different types of hair shafts. Terminal hairs are large and pigmented in young individuals. Small, unpigmented hairs are called vellus hairs. There are hairs intermediate in caliber and length between the two types called indeterminate hairs. A brief review of hair cycling, which all hairs follicles continue throughout the lifetime of an individual, will aid in conceptualizing several conditions discussed in this chapter. Some types of hair loss from the scalp can be characterized by alterations in growth cycles.

Hair follicle activity is intermittent and characterized by a growth phase (anagen), followed by a brief transition phase (catagen) and a resting phase (telogen). Normally 90% or more of scalp hair is in the anagen phase at any given time, 10% or less is in the telogen phase and less than 1% is in catagen. The anagen phase is determined genetically and differs in individuals. The length of the anagen phase determines the natural length an individual's hair will attain and tends to remain stable unless pathologic alterations intervene. Telogen hairs are also retained for a defined period of time and then shed. On the scalp, telogen hairs are held 2–3 months before they are shed. The follicles in different anatomic sites vary in duration of anagen and telogen phase, which gives hair its growth characteristics by site. Those areas with long anagen cycles and a short telogen phase, such as scalp hair, produce a long fiber. A short anagen growth phase, coupled with a prolonged telogen phase, produces the shorter, stable hairs of the eyebrows and eyelashes, and the terminal hairs on the extremities. Scalp hair grows at approximately one centimeter a month, although the growth rate slows down with advanced age.

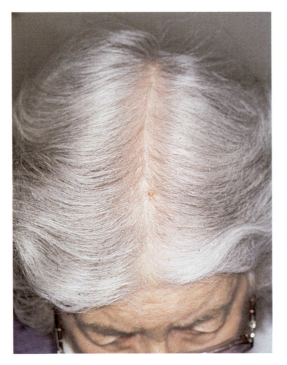

Figure 5 Vertex view of 86-year-old woman with senescent alopecia

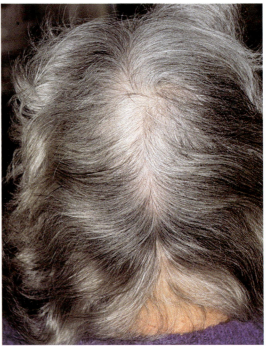

Figure 6 Occipital view of the same woman as in Figure 5

Hair shafts and root sheaths are of ectodermal derivation. The dermal papillae that nourish the follicles are mesodermal in origin. Because hair follicles are self-renewing, they contain a population of slow-cycling stem cells. The stem cells of hair follicles are thought to be located at the 'bulge' region in the outer root sheath near the insertion of the arrector pili muscle[16]. Cotsarelis and colleagues suggested that the anagen phase is initiated when stem cells are activated by signals from the dermal papilla[16]. This has implications in scarring versus non-scarring hair conditions, which will be addressed in the following sections.

Scalp hair loss can result from scarring or permanent destruction of the follicles, disturbance of the respective hair cycles and changes in follicular architecture.

SENESCENT ALOPECIA

Etiology

Follicular density decreases with age (Table 1)[17]. This process is called senescent or involutional alopecia and is defined as global or diffuse hair thinning, without vertex accentuation, after 50 years of age. Vertex and occipital regions are similarly affected. It is a result of a reduction in follicle size and alterations in hair cycling. Both sexes can be affected. These losses reflect follicular dropout, which is not a scarring process, but rather a process in which hair follicles gradually cease to produce a hair shaft. This may be a result of exhaustion of the allocated anagen-telogen cycles within an individual's life span, which is perhaps genetically predetermined and appears to be highly variable. Life events which 'use up' or accelerate these cycles may alter the age of onset and extent of senescent alopecia. Some octogenarians have remarkably dense hair. Other individuals demonstrate an obvious global decrease in hair density in the sixth decade. The androgen-dependent hair of the extremities and pubic and axillary regions may diminish in the postmenopausal female as a result of diminishing androgen production.

Table 1 Follicular density by age

Age	Approximate number of hairs/cm²
Birth	1135
1 year	795
15 years	615
30 years+	485
80 years	435

Table reproduced with permission from Olsen E. *Disorders of Hair Growth, Diagnosis and Treatment*. New York: McGraw Hill

Histopathology

Histopathology shows an increase in numbers of telogen follicles and a decrease in follicle size, perhaps reflecting a decrease in volume of actively dividing matrix cells in the hair bulb[18,19].

Diagnosis

The diagnosis can generally be made clinically by evaluating the entire head. If density is diminished globally with no patchy hair loss or evidence of scarring, a presumptive diagnosis can be made. Compare the part width on the vertex and occiput; in senescent alopecia, they are the same or nearly so (Figures 5 and 6).

Treatment

There are no available data on therapy for senescent alopecia. Anecdotal reports of scalp hair regrowth in elderly individuals using oral minoxidil provide a rationale for the trial of topical minoxidil. See treatment section of androgenetic alopecia for details. Much remains to be clarified regarding the incidence, etiology and pathophysiology of senescent hair loss.

TELOGEN EFFLUVIUM

Hair matrix cells are among the most rapidly proliferating cells in the body, second only to bone marrow cells. Consequently numerous physiologic insults may result in an increase in the premature transformation of anagen to telogen hairs. Simultaneous cycling of numerous anagen hairs into the telogen phase results in increasing numbers of telogen or 'club' hairs shed daily. This phenomenon is called telogen effluvium[20]. On the normal scalp 50–100 hairs are shed daily and fall relatively unnoticed by the individual. Effluvium is Latin for 'to flow out' and aptly describes the fall of telogen hairs. Hair is shed diffusely from all over the scalp, although the temples and anterior hairline tend to be more severely affected[18]. This suggests diverse mechanisms of telogen effluvium and Headington[21] defined five functional types based on changes in different phases of the follicular cycle. The type relevant to physiologic insult is called 'immediate anagen release' and results from follicles prematurely entering the telogen phase. Regrowth follows cessation of the insult and resumption of normal follicular cycling. Normal density is regained provided senescent alopecia or androgenetic alopecia is not unmasked.

Disturbances in normal cycling occur in response to numerous insults. Postpartum hair loss[22,23], nutritional causes including protein and iron deficiency[5,24], and oral contraceptive use predominate in the premenopausal female. Telogen effluvium in younger males is uncommon.

The causes of telogen effluvium are different in the postmenopausal female and older male patient (Table 2). The incidence increases for events associated more with aging, such as acute[25] and chronic illnesses, surgery and the use of medications for all manner of conditions[26]. Figure 7 shows regrowing hair after telogen effluvium following surgery. Note that a dark background helps to visualize the tips of the regrowing hair. Insufficient dietary protein may pose a problem in the elderly when issues of ill health, deficiencies of self-care and social isolation may become manifest[27]. Telogen effluvium may result when thyroid replacement requirements decrease in the postmenopausal female. Hair shedding may be the first symptom of changing thyroid status[28–30]. Iron deficiency is not as prevalent as the chronic iron losses due to menstruation cease

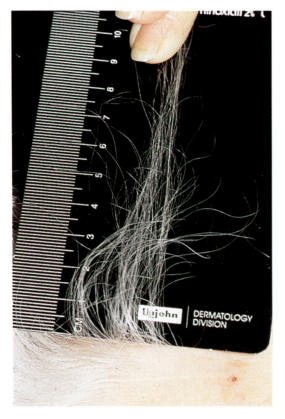

Figure 7 Regrowth of hair following post-surgery telogen effluvium. Note that visualization of regrowing tapered hair tips is facilitated by dark background

Table 2   Causes of telogen effluvium

Premenopausal females	Hypothyroidism
	Hyperthyroidism
	Iron deficiency
	Oral contraceptives
	Sudden weight loss
	Protein deficiency
Older males and females	Acute illness
	Chronic illness
	Surgery
	Anesthesia
	Drugs
	Iron deficiency
	Protein deficiency

(unpublished data, Roberts JL). Zinc deficiency and essential free fatty acid deficiency, common in the 1970s and 1980s in patients on total parenteral nutrition, has been largely eliminated in the West as knowledge about nutrition requirements has improved[31-33]. Fewer older individuals undergo the stresses of rapid weight loss due to intentional 'crash dieting' but may suffer unintentional weight loss due to various illnesses. Chronic illnesses and dietary deficiencies can both result in lowered serum albumin.

The number of drugs reported to cause telogen effluvium is large[26,34]. The *Physician's Desk Reference* and *Drug: Facts and Comparisons* list alopecia occurring between 1% and 2% of the time for many drugs. These statistics relate to reports of telogen effluvium during clinical trials or post-marketing reporting. In the author's experience, confirmed by reports in the literature, several drugs are commonly associated with increased hair shedding and deserve special mention. Among these are beta-blockers, both oral and intraocular, antihyperlipemic drugs, non-steroidal anti-inflammatory drugs and anticoagulants. Antimitotic drugs result in anagen effluvium (see following section), although low doses may cause telogen effluvium. Table 3 lists drugs that may be implicated in shedding.

The paradox of hormone replacement in postmenopausal females should be considered. Estrogen prolongs the anagen phase, increases sex-steroid-binding globulin and, hence, may be helpful in preventing the accelerated expression of androgenetic alopecia and/or senescent alopecia that occurs in many women postmenopausally. Progesterone may be androgenic and contribute to androgenetic alopecia. Progesterone and estrogen have both been reported to cause shedding. Hence, estrogen and progesterone may be both beneficial and detrimental. Acute or chronic telogen effluvium may unmask or accelerate the expression of androgenetic alopecia or senescent alopecia in genetically prone individuals.

Whiting in 1996 reported on the clinical and histopathology criteria for a type of idiopathic telogen effluvium in middle-aged women. These women are typically 30–60 years of age and complain of generalized diffuse thinning all over the scalp rather than

Table 3   Drugs that may cause hair loss

Antibiotics	*Antihypertensive agents*	Hydroxyurea	*Histamine (H2) antagonists*
Ethambutol	Atenolol	Interferon	Cimetidine
Ethionamide	Captopril	Methotrexate	Famotidine
Gentamycin	Enalapril	Radiation	Ranitidine
Nitrofurantoin	Labetalol	Vincristine	*Hormones*
Streptomycin	Metoprolol	*Antipsychotic agents*	Anabolic steroids
Anticoagulants	Minoxidil	All tricyclic antidepressants	Clomiphene
Bishydroxycoumarin	Nadolol	Benzodiazepines	Corticosteroids
Coumarin	Propranolol	Buspirone HCl	Danazol
Dextran	Verapamil	Clomipramine HCl	Oral contraceptives
Gemfibrozil	*Intraocular*	Doxepin HCl	Progesterones
Heparin	Betaxolol	Fluoxetine	*Miscellaneous drugs*
Heparinoids	Levobunolol	Fluvoxamine	Acyclovir
Anticonvulsants	Timolol	Lithium	Amphetamines
Carbamazepine	*Anti-inflammatory agents*	Paroxetine HCl	Boric acid
Clonazopam	Diclofenac	Phenothiazines	Bromocriptine
Trimethadione	Ibuprofen	Sertraline HCl	Diethylpropion HCl
Valproic acid	Indomethacin	Trazodone	Hydroxychloroquine sulfate
Antifungal agents	Naproxen	*Antithyroid drugs*	Levodopa
Fluconazole	Piroxicam	Carbimazole	Methysergide
Itraconazole	Salicylates	Iodine	Nifedipine
Terbinafine	Sulindac	Methylthiouracil	Penicillamine
Antigout agents	*Antikeratinizing agents*	Propylthiouracil	Pyridostigmine
Allopurinol	Etretinate	*Heavy metals*	Quinacrine
Probenecid	Isotretinoin	Arsenic	Spironolactone
Colchicine	Thallium	Bismuth	Sulfasalazine
Antihyperlipidemic agents	Vitamin A	Gold	Alendronate
Simvastatin	*Antimitotic agents*	Lead	
Lovastatin	Alkaloids	Mercury	
Pravastatin	Alkylating drugs	Selenium	
Fluvastatin	Antimetabolites		
Atorvastatin	Colchicine		
Niacin	Cyclophosphamide		

vertex accentuation. The onset is abrupt, with a fluctuating course. No etiology can be determined. Histopathology is distinctive[35].

Evaluation

Working with the patient's primary care physician is particularly important in the geriatric population as health issues become more complex. Very careful health and medication history is imperative. A careful dietary history needs to be assessed to ensure that there is adequate caloric and protein intake. Notes of any acute and chronic health problems and medications used, including prescription and over-the-counter medications, should be made. The timing of new medications should be noted in relationship to the onset of shedding. Generally the initiation of drug therapy can be timed to the duration of the telogen phase, resulting in a lag period of 2–3 months before the onset of shedding. Cause and effect of drug therapy should be carefully documented, if possible, with particular attention paid to the onset of shedding and cessation of shedding, which follows 2 to 3 months after the discontinuation of a specific medication (dechallenge). If appropriate, rechallenge with the suspected medication may be helpful. Particular attention should be given to thyroid evaluation and replacement therapy. Patients can shed from over-replacement as well as under-replacement of thyroid.

A careful counting of the hairs shed over a three-day or weekly period will help establish the diagnosis, if telogen hair shedding averages over 100/day. Physical examination of the scalp and hair should be performed to rule out scarring or patchy hair loss. Light hair pull is considered positive if 2–3 hairs are retrieved on freshly shampooed hair or 5–6 hairs on unwashed hair. Visualization of the regrowing hair tips will help to determine the length of hairs growing, which can be a helpful clue in determining the onset of shedding. Generally the hair begins to regrow at the time of shedding and grows a fairly consistent one centimeter a month.

Laboratory tests should be based on the historical findings. A chemical screening battery should be obtained for evidence of specific chronic diseases, including thyroid stimulating hormone deficiency. Lowered serum albumin may be detected if dietary protein is deficient or the patient is chronically ill. Carry out an antinuclear antibody (ANA) screen if an autoimmune disorder is suspected. The assessment of hematocrit and hemoglobin is not sufficient, as iron stores may be depleted in spite of normal values. For the assessment of the adequacy of iron, some clinicians rely on serum iron and per cent saturation. Others prefer to monitor ferritin levels as an indicator of total body iron stores. Because ferritin is an acute phase reactant, it is important to obtain an erythrocyte sedimentation rate (ESR) as well. If ESR is elevated, the ferritin is usually artificially elevated. Rushton and Ramsay have suggested that ferritin levels should be at least 40 µg/dl, if not higher, to ensure adequate stores for regrowth of hair and as a basis for response to therapy for androgenetic alopecia[36]. Iron is an essential element in several enzyme systems related to hair growth.

Treatment

The prognosis for spontaneous hair regrowth is good if the underlying causes are addressed, provided senescent and/or androgenetic alopecia is not unmasked or accelerated. In the older age groups, however, chronic diseases and illnesses of aging make chronic telogen effluvium more common. Any dietary deficiencies should be corrected. Iron replacement is necessary in those individuals deficient on testing. If the patient is on thyroid replacement therapy, it should be finely tuned. At times, it is not possible to substitute with a drug that will not cause shedding. This is particularly true of hyperlipemic drugs, many of which can cause shedding. Beta-blockers used orally for hypertension and intraocularly for glaucoma present another dilemma, as most of the drugs in this class have been reported to cause shedding[37–39]. The anticoagulants heparin and coumadin have both been implicated in shedding, leaving little choice but to tolerate the side-effects[40]. The choice of medications used to treat osteoporosis is limited; they have been reported to cause telogen effluvium.

ANAGEN EFFLUVIUM

Anagen effluvium is the shedding of anagen or growing hairs following common therapeutic doses of chemotherapeutic drugs or radiation, usually for the treatment of cancer. Because 90% or more of scalp hair is typically in the anagen phase at any given time, up to 90% of hair may be lost as the hair shafts are attenuated by the abrupt interference with, or cessation of, mitosis in the hair matrix. Hair matrix cells are especially vulnerable to the effects of toxic drugs and radiation because they are so metabolically active, dividing on average every 9–12 hours. Shedding generally begins within days to a few weeks after therapy as the attenuated hair shafts reach the surface of the scalp. The 10% of hairs not lost in the immediate 2–3 weeks post therapy are probably telogen hairs that will be shed as a natural event, rendering the loss of scalp hair virtually complete in many patients. If the insult is temporary, as in the case of intermittent or episodic therapy, regrowth should be virtually complete because the bulge area has not been subjected to injury. As discussed in the introduction, this side-effect may be the most traumatic one that cancer patients endure.

Treatment

No treatment is necessary for hair to regrow once therapy is terminated. The issue of cooling of the scalp to prevent hair loss is controversial. Cooling devices have been developed which can help some patients avoid this consequence of chemotherapy by cooling the scalp during administration of the drugs and for one hour following. Controversy surrounds this technique, with advocates and detractors, both those who feel it is not beneficial enough to warrant use and those who feel that scalp metastases remain a risk to the patient[3]. Robinson and colleagues in 1987 reported scalp cooling to be effective in preventing hair loss in breast cancer therapy with epirubicin as mono-therapy[41]. Ron and co-workers in 1997 reported treating 35 breast cancer patients with a scalp cooling device while administering doxorubicin, cyclophosphamide and 5-flurouracil[42]. Forty-eight per cent of those with cooling suffered anagen effluvium, compared to 81% without the cooling treatment. They reported no scalp metastases in follow-up. Tollenaar and colleagues[43] found that only 11% had acceptable hair loss prevention; 34% had moderate preservation, but still needed to wear a wig; 54% had complete hair loss. They, too, reported no scalp metastases, but concluded that, with the current regimen of drugs given, the benefits are not substantial enough to warrant the procedure.

ANDROGENETIC ALOPECIA

Clinical presentation

Scalp, facial, pubic, axillary and body hair follicles in different regions are variably responsive to androgens, especially testosterone and dihydrotestosterone. Pubic and axillary hair transforms from vellus to terminal hair in response to modest levels of testosterone. Facial and body hair growth requires the 5α-reduced product of testosterone, dihydrotestosterone, for expression[44]. Androgenetic alopecia is the androgen-dependent miniaturization of scalp hair in genetically susceptible men and women. It involves long-term changes in follicular architecture and alterations of growth cycles. Paradoxically, androgenetic alopecia in both males and females results from a reversion of terminal hairs back to hairs smaller in caliber and shorter in length as a response to dihydrotestosterone. Hair follicles are not only capable of responding to androgens, but are capable of participating in the metabolism of androgens. This peripheral metabolism of hormones contributes significantly to the overall endocrine system.

The potential length a hair will grow is determined by the duration of the anagen phase. The volume of matrix cells in the hair bulb, which produce the hair shaft, determines the diameter. Miniaturization is the result of shortening of the duration of anagen and decrease in the volume of matrix cells[45]. Figure 8 depicts the miniaturizing effect of androgens on scalp hair. Males tend to exhibit uniform miniaturization in genetically predetermined patterns. Females tend to have a predominance of decrease in the matrix volume while maintaining a relative longer anagen period of growth, resulting in hair with relatively longer shafts but very fine in caliber (Figure 9).

It is estimated that 50% or more of Caucasian males and females have some degree of androgenetic alopecia by age 50 years. Androgenetic alopecia in males and females has different, but familiar phenotypes[46]. Males express the various patterns of vertex hair loss classified by Hamilton[47] and later modified by Norwood (Figure 10)[48]. Females have more diffuse loss over the vertex with retention of the frontal hairline. Approximately 5% of males express the female phenotype[49].

Many females suffer an initial or further decrease in vertex density at menopause. Venning and Dawber reported on a clinical study of 564 hormonally normal women and found that 13% of premenopausal women and 37% of postmenopausal women had frontal and fronto-parietal recession, respectively[50]. They concluded that patterned hair loss is more common than described, particularly in postmenopausal women. See Figure 11 which pictures an elderly female with a dramatic difference between the vertex and occipital part-width.

Etiology

Hamilton demonstrated that androgens are a prerequisite for the expression of androgenetic alopecia in males[47]. Testosterone is converted to dihydrotestosterone (DHT) by the enzyme 5α-reductase of which there are two types, designated type I and type II. In the 1970s observations of male pseudohermaphrodites lacking the enzyme type II 5α-reductase further defined the role of hormones in the development of androgenetic alopecia. These individuals, who do not develop androgenetic alopecia, demonstrated that dihydrotestosterone, rather that testosterone, is the hormone responsible for the development of androgenetic alopecia in men[51]. Type II 5α-reductase predominates in scalp hair follicles whereas type I 5α-reductase predominates

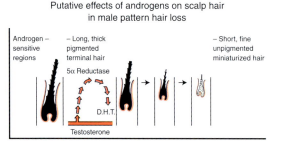

Figure 8 Miniaturizing effect of androgens on scalp hair. Figure reproduced with permission from Wade M, Sinclair R. Disorders of hair. In Parish LC, Brenner S, Ramos-e-Silva M, eds. *Women's Dermatology*. London: Parthenon Publishing 2000;137

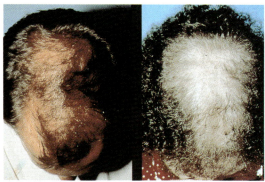

Figure 9 Male (left) and female with androgenetic alopecia. Male has definable pattern, while female shows diffuse decrease in hair density over scalp vertex

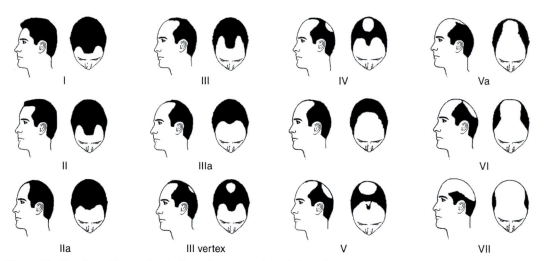

Figure 10   Hamilton–Norwood scale for androgenetic alopecia in males

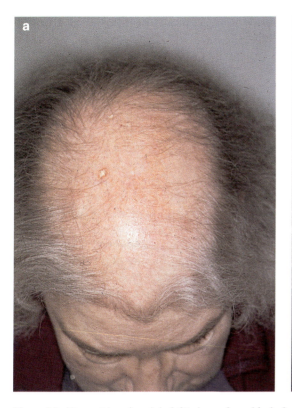 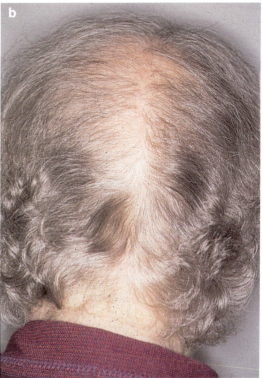

Figure 11 Vertex (a) and occipital (b) views of an elderly female with a dramatic variation in part width

in scalp skin. Testosterone is the major precursor of dihydrotestosterone in men.

The pathophysiology of androgenetic alopecia in females is less well defined. In women, 50–60% of testosterone and dihydrotestosterone is produced by peripheral conversion of weaker androgens such as dehydroepiandrosterone. Sawaya and Price[52] demonstrated consistent differences in hair follicles from young women and men with and without androgenetic alopecia. With reference to type II 5α-reductase, young females and males with androgenetic alopecia have higher levels of types I and II 5α-reductase in frontal hair follicles than occipital follicles. Androgen receptor content is 40% lower on the frontal scalp of females with androgenetic alopecia than males. Aromatase, responsible for converting testosterone and dihydrotestosterone back to estradiol, is six times more plentiful on female scalps. It is postulated that the higher levels of aromatase found in females may be responsible for the phenotypic differences and less severe expression of androgenetic alopecia in females[52].

It is not known at present if these same distinctions prevail in individuals over 50 years of age with androgenetic alopecia. Whether the menopausal and postmenopausal acceleration of androgenetic alopecia in women relates to a reduction in estrogen production, changes in adrenal androgen production with relative androgen dominance, or is the result of senescent effects, is unclear.

Diagnosis

The diagnosis of androgenetic alopecia in men and women can be made clinically by examining the entire scalp to rule out patchy hair loss or scarring. In women, compare the part width over the vertex with the occipital scalp. The part width will be wider over the vertex. In senescent alopecia, they are the same.

Treatment

Recent studies with 1 mg finasteride, a pure type II 5α-reductase inhibitor, have shown that it increases hair count and slows progression of androgenetic alopecia in 83% of males aged 18–41 years as measured by total hair count, increased percentage of anagen hairs in a target area[53], global photographic assessment and investigator and subject assessment, with the effect maintained over two years[54]. Finasteride reduces serum dihydrotestosterone levels by 67%. Finasteride (Propecia®) was FDA approved in early 1998 for the treatment of men aged 18–41 years with androgenetic alopecia. The effect of finasteride on males 41–60 years old with androgenetic alopecia is currently being evaluated. A 1-year double-blind, placebo-controlled study using 1 mg finasteride in postmenopausal females 41–59 years of age with androgenetic alopecia yielded negative results. Treated and placebo groups both showed a slight net loss in hair count in the target area at one year[55].

The mechanism of action of minoxidil, first formulated as an oral antihypertensive agent, on hair follicles is not clearly understood. Hypertrichosis was an unanticipated and serendipitous side-effect. Minoxidil is a vasodilator that works on vascular smooth muscle by opening potassium channels. Uno and colleagues[56] have done extensive research with minoxidil on the stump-tailed macaque, a primate which has long served as the primary animal model for androgenetic alopecia. They observed early on that minoxidil both grossly and microscopically enlarges vellus follicles to the size of mid-sized and terminal follicles (regrowth) and maintains terminal follicles in prebalding scalps (prevention). The earlier treatment was instituted the better the response of therapy. They further showed that minoxidil enhances DNA synthesis in follicular but not epidermal keratinocytes[56]. It causes proliferation and

differentiation of the matrix cells in the hair bulb[57].

Two per cent minoxidil has been available for a number of years for the treatment of males and females under the age of 49 with androgenetic alopecia[58]. A 5% topical solution of minoxidil (Rogaine Extra Strength for Men®) was granted FDA approval in 1997 for treatment of men. Approval was not granted for use of the 5% solution in females, for lack of clear benefit over the 2% solution. The efficacy of topical minoxidil has not been evaluated in males and females over 50 years of age. Therapeutic trial in individuals over 50 years is warranted because of the observation of hair regrowth following the use of oral minoxidil.

Topical antiandrogens such as progesterone and estrogen have not been systematically evaluated in females of any age. The use of systemic antiandrogens such as spironolactone, flutamide and cimetidine is precluded in males because of the potential sexual side-effects. Value in the treatment of androgenetic alopecia in pre- and postmenopausal women has not been documented in carefully conducted trials[49]. There remain many facets of androgenetic alopecia and the relationship to senescent alopecia yet to be determined.

Clinical correlations

The possible correlation between baldness and coronary artery disease has been explored in a number of epidemiologic studies on men[59–64]. No similar studies have been reported for women. Trevisan and colleagues reported on 872 factory workers in southern Italy, comparing cholesterol levels and blood pressure with type of balding[62]. They looked at those men who had no balding, frontotemporal recession only (M-shaped resculpturing in postadolescent males) compared with men who had frontotemporal and occipital (vertex) loss. A positive correlation was found with the more severe phenotype and elevated cholesterol and younger age. The relationship became weaker in older individuals. There was no correlation between age and balding with blood pressure. Results indicate that a vertex pattern of baldness is associated with an elevated risk profile for coronary heart disease, and the relationship between age and serum cholesterol differs in younger compared to older men.

Also in 1993, Lesko and co-workers[59] reported on a case–controlled, hospital-based study of 655 men between the ages of 21 and 54 who were experiencing their first myocardial infarction. They were age-matched with patients admitted to the hospital for non-cardiac related illnesses with no prior history of any cardiac disorder. They found that frontal balding was not associated with an increased risk of myocardial infarction, while vertex balding was associated with an increased risk and that this risk increased with the extent of balding. There was an almost three-fold risk with severe vertex balding (1.3 versus 3.4).

In 1997 Ford and colleagues[60] reported similar findings on 3932 men who were rated as having none, minimal, moderate and severe balding. The cohort was followed for 14 years. For men under age 55 at baseline, there was a positive correlation between severe baldness and ischemic heart disease and mortality. The authors hypothesized that there may be some mechanistic relationship between male pattern balding and ischemic heart disease.

The Framingham study, reported by Herrera and colleagues[61] in 1995, followed a cohort of males for up to 30 years. They looked at the progression of balding for new coronary heart-related death, cardiovascular disease and death from any cause. The extent of baldness was not associated with any outcome. Progression of the balding pattern, however, was associated with coronary heart disease occurrence, mortality and all-cause mortality, concluding that rapid hair loss may be a marker for coronary heart disease.

Two studies finding no associated risk between coronary artery disease and baldness are worthy of note. Halim and co-workers studied 48 men who had recovered from myocardial infarction and age-matched controls[63]. No evidence was found in relationship to androgenic stimulation, assessing plasma testosterone, muscle thickness, sebum excretion rate, androgenetic alopecia or density of terminal hair on the body. There was a slight increase in muscle and bone thickness. Cooke[64] studied 478 male in-patient Caucasians, finding no correlation with coronary artery disease and male pattern alopecia, premature male pattern alopecia or male pattern alopecia with a positive family history. Men with hypertension, diabetes mellitus or elevated cholesterol levels were excluded from the study.

Histopathology

The first pathologic change noted in early biopsies of androgenetic alopecia is degeneration of the lower third of the connective tissue sheath around the growing or anagen hair follicles. As the condition becomes more severe, the histology mirrors the clinical picture: that of progressive miniaturization of affected terminal hair follicles in a mosaic pattern[65]. The diminution of the follicle size is accompanied by shortening of the anagen phase[57]. The connective tissue sheath is replaced by a 'streamer' underneath the miniaturized follicles. The miniaturized anagen hairs retain the arrector pili muscle in contrast with true vellus hairs, which are also found in increased numbers. Similarly the percent of telogen hairs increase, probably as a result of shortening of the anagen phase. Young and colleagues[66] reported granular deposits of IgM or C3 or both at the basement membrane of 96% of specimens from involved scalps as well as porphyrins, possibly from the action of UV radiation on *Propionibacterium acnes* around the follicles. Lattanand and Johnson found a moderate amount of chronic inflammatory cells surrounding capillaries and adnexal structures[67]. Both of these authors believe that the androgenetic effect is an inflammatory process. Macguire and Kligman noted no such association in 1962[65]. However, Jaworsky, Kligman and Murphy in 1992 examined the ultrastructural changes in alopetic scalp skin, noting progressive fibrosis of the perifollicular sheath associated with mast cell degranulation and fibroblast activation, predated by T-cell infiltration of follicular stem cell epithelium. Injury to follicular stem cell epithelium and/or thickening of the advential sheaths may impair normal hair cycling and lead to hair loss[68].

SCARRING ALOPECIA

Scarring or permanent alopecia can present a confusing clinical picture. Early diagnosis and treatment are essential. Scarring is the result of destruction of the stem cells at the region of the bulge. Once a hair follicle has been destroyed, it is irretrievably lost. Patients presenting with patchy or ill-defined hair loss should be examined thoroughly for any signs of scarring as manifested by patchy hair loss, obliteration of follicular orifices, signs of inflammation – erythema, telangiectasias, follicular hyperkeratosis, or pigmentary changes. The remainder of the skin, mucous membranes and nails should be examined, looking for signs of lichen planus or discoid lupus erythematosus.

If scarring is present or suspected, early biopsy is important, and ideally should include two 4 mm biopsies, one for either vertical or horizontal sectioning stained with hematoxylin and eosin, and a second one for immunofluorescent evaluation[69,70]. A periodic acid-Schiff (PAS) stain may be helpful in examining basement membrane thickening (as may be noted in lupus erythematosus), catagen hairs for apoptotic cells (as commonly seen in trichotillomania) and fungal organisms (if tinea capitis is suspected).

Scarring or permanent alopecias can be divided into inflammatory and non-inflammatory types[71]. Non-inflammatory causes include hereditary, developmental and neoplastic tumors, both benign and malignant. Of these, those causes that are developmental and hereditary will most probably be expressed and, hence, diagnosed before the geriatric age group under consideration in this chapter. Neoplastic lesions can be either primary to the scalp or metastatic to the scalp. Of the malignant tumors that are primary to the scalp, basal cell carcinoma and squamous cell carcinomas are common. Malignant melanoma and malignant hamartomas can be primary to the scalp. Both B-cell and T-cell lymphomas may occur on the scalp. Cutaneous T-cell lymphoma (CTCL) may exhibit a tendency to affect the follicles preferentially. Alopecia mucinosa occurs either in association with CTCL or primary to the scalp.

Of lesions metastatic to the scalp, the most common primaries are to be found in the breast, kidney and lung. Papillary thyroid carcinoma metastasizing to the scalp is commonly reported in the literature. There are many reports in the literature of a multiplicity of different common and rare malignant tumors presenting initially as scalp nodules. Any lesion that is new, grows rapidly or appears unfamiliar, especially in the geriatric age group, should be biopsied.

Inflammatory scarring alopecias include discoid lupus erythematosus, lichen planopilaris, folliculitis decalvans and infectious processes. Four scarring alopecias deserve special mention as they are nearly unique to middle-aged and older women: frontal fibrosing alopecia, erosive pustular dermatosis, follicular degeneration syndrome and pseudopelade of Brocq. Frontal fibrosing alopecia has been reported exclusively in postmenopausal females. Erosive pustular dermatosis was first reported in elderly females. Follicular degeneration syndrome is typically seen in middle-aged black females. A more recent study reports the occurrence in middle-aged black males. Pseudopelade of Brocq primarily affects adult females.

FRONTAL FIBROSING ALOPECIA

In 1994 Kossard reported the occurrence of a frontal scarring alopecia associated with perifollicular erythema in the frontal and parietal marginal hairline in six postmenopausal women[72]. None had skin or mucous membrane lesions suggestive of lichen planus. Hormonal studies showed no elevation of systemic androgens. He theorized that this type of follicular destruction could possibly be a reaction pattern triggered by events underlying the frontal hairline recession seen in postmenopausal females. Feldmann, Harmes and Saurat in 1996 reported two females with frontal fibrosing alopecia characterized by progressive recession of the fronto-temporal and parietal hair margins, leading to a margin of scarring 3–6 centimeters wide[73]. One of their patients also had vulvar lichen sclerosis et atrophicus. Lee and colleagues subsequently described a 52-year-old postmenopausal female with similar clinical findings[74]. Trueb and Torricelli, in a 1998 article[75], described a 68-year-old woman with frontal fibrosing alopecia and lesions of the buccal mucosa typical of lichen planus, and suggested the possibility that the condition could actually represent a variation of lichen planopilaris with a predilection for the frontal hairline. Kossard, Lee and Wilkinson refined their initial report in a 1997 article reporting on 16 postmenopausal women, with clinical findings consistent with Kossard's 1994 article, adding that 13 of these women also suffered a total or marked decrease in eyebrows. They compared the histology of the frontal fibrosing variety with multifocal lichen planopilaris and found it indistinguishable. They concluded that postmenopausal frontal fibrosing alopecia is a distinct variant of lichen planopilaris often affecting the eyebrows as well[76].

Treatment

Feldmann and colleagues[73] indicated that there is no known treatment but that the disease seems to be self-limiting. Kossard and co-workers report treatment attempts with oral steroids and antimalarials, which they found may slow the progression of the disease; hormonal replacement did not alter its course[76].

Histopathology

Histopathology is indistinguishable from that of lichen planopilaris. See following section.

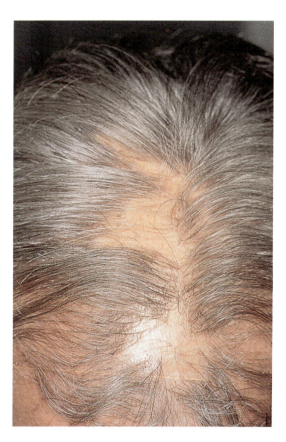

Figure 12   Scarring alopecia (lichen planopilaris)

MULTIFOCAL LICHEN PLANOPILARIS

Lichen planopilaris generally presents as multifocal areas of patchy scarring alopecia in middle-aged adults, women being more often affected[77]. Lesions tend to expand and coalesce and show perifollicular erythema, follicular hyperkeratosis and follicular plugging (Figure 12). Half of the patients have or develop lesions of lichen planus on the skin and mucous membranes or nails.

Histopathology

The histopathology consists of prominent perifollicular lymphocytic infiltration, often band-like; fibrosis centered around the isthmus and infundibular areas of the follicles; and an increase in apoptosis of the keratinocytes.

Cytoid bodies may be located near the follicular epithelium. Direct immunofluorescence shows globular IgM within the dermis adjacent to follicular epithelium[78]. Cytoid bodies stain with anti-IgM and anti-IgA[77]. Immunotyping of lymphocytes shows a dominance of activated helper T cells with no difference between frontal fibrosing alopecia and multifocal lichen planopilaris. The histopathology is indistinguishable from that of postmenopausal frontal fibrosing alopecia. See above section.

Treatment

Oral and topical corticosteroids and antimalarial drugs are the mainstay of therapy. Oral isotretinoin and etretinate have shown a benefit.

EROSIVE PUSTULAR DERMATOSIS

In 1979 Pye and colleagues reported on a previously undescribed entity characterized by expanding round to oval patches with peripheral pustules and crusts rapidly leading to scarring[79]. All six patients were elderly females. Several reports have subsequently been published confirming this as a distinct entity[80–82]. However, it has been suggested that trauma may play a role in etiology. Cases have included surgical scalp excision and grafting[83], traumatic avulsion of the scalp[83], post-trigeminal herpes zoster infection[84] and malnutrition in young African patients[85]. In all reports, the bacterial, mycological and viral cultures were negative. Watanbe and co-workers report the association with Hashimoto's thyroiditis, aortitis, and autoimmune hepatitis and speculate on a common autoimmune pathogenesis[81].

Clinical presentation

Erosive pustular dermatosis is characterized by round to oval patches of alopecia that are smooth, with no signs of inflammation in the center of the patches. Around the periphery are follicular pustules which occur in crops (Figure 13).

Treatment

Those cases reported by Pye's group did not respond to oral antibiotics, but were suppressed by potent topical steroids[79]. The other reports concur, using both oral and topical steroids. Wollenberg and colleagues reported a good therapeutic response to oral zinc[84].

Histopathology

The histopathology is non-diagnostic in all cases, showing only non-specific changes of chronic inflammation and sometimes increased plasma cells, spongiform pustule formation[82] and atrophy and destruction of hair follicles[79,86].

FOLLICULAR DEGENERATION SYNDROME

In 1992 Sperling and Sau[87] reported on the clinical findings, history and histologic findings in 10 middle-aged black women with a distinctive, common scarring alopecia that had previously been called 'hot comb alopecia'. Scarring tended to be progressive and localized primarily over the vertex of the scalp. Patients were carefully queried about their hair-care habits. There was little correlation between the use of hot combs and onset or progression of scarring. Sperling and colleagues[88] extended this description to a series of 8 black male patients who had no association with chemical or mechanical styling practices.

Treatment

There are no suggested treatments available to alter the course of this disease process.

Histopathology

Sperling's group studied both transverse and vertical biopsy specimens in females and males. Transverse biopsies showed premature desquamation of the internal root sheath as the earliest observable abnormality, followed by events leading to complete destruction of the follicle: thinning of the outer root sheath with a mononuclear infiltrate, degeneration and eventual destruction of the follicular epithelium leaving the hair fiber free in the dermis. This leads to hair fiber granuloma formation and replacement of the follicle with a thick, fibrous tract. Histology in both sexes is identical.

INFLAMMATORY SCALP DISORDERS

Three inflammatory scalp disorders deserve discussion: psoriasis, seborrheic dermatitis and dermatomyositis. Psoriasis of the scalp and seborrheic dermatitis are both common in older individuals. Seborrheic dermatitis can be aggravated by associated neurologic disorders. Psoriasis is difficult to manage especially for geriatric patients by themselves. Dermatomyositis of the scalp may mimic seborrheic dermatitis and be a cutaneous marker for internal disease that is particularly associated with internal malignancies and, hence, more common in the geriatric population.

SEBORRHEIC DERMATITIS

Seborrheic dermatitis is characterized by greasy, yellowish scales distributed diffusely over the scalp. Areas of predilection include the hairline, retroauricular and posterior neck, beard, nasolabial folds, eyebrows, sternum and groin (Figure 14). It is accompanied by variable degrees of inflammation. When severe, seborrheic dermatitis may be accompanied by mild to moderate telogen effluvium.

The incidence and severity may be increased in patients with Parkinson's disease, cerebrovascular accidents[89], head trauma and epilepsy[90–92]. These neurologic disorders may be implicated in exacerbating seborrheic dermatitis by increasing sebum rates, although there is no direct correlation between sebum production and seborrheic dermatitis.

Etiology

Pityrosporum ovale may contribute to the pathogenesis of seborrheic dermatitis[93–94]. The density of *P. ovale* organisms has been correlated with the clinical severity. The metabolism of *P. ovale*-generated free fatty acids may contribute to the inflammatory process. Cause and effect are uncertain. Neuber and colleagues reported results supporting the assumption that strong colonization with *P. ovale* in seborrheic dermatitis is due to altered cellular immunity, which may be induced by increased interleukin-10 (IL-10) secretion[93].

Histopathology

The stratum corneum shows focal parakeratosis. The epidermis shows mild to moderate acanthosis and spongiosis with mononuclear cells contained within the spongiotic areas. There is a mild mononuclear infiltrate in the dermis.

Treatment

Treatment must be directed towards both scale removal, reduction of inflammation and reduction of *P. ovale* organisms. The frequency of shampooing is important, with daily to alternate daily shampooing ideal. This may prove difficult to accomplish for some older individuals, either through physical limitations and lack of compliance due to more set shampooing regimens for those patients having to rely on health aides or hair stylists for help with shampooing.

Tar shampoos address the scale formation secondary to epidermal proliferation. They are a mechanism to apply medication and should not necessarily be considered a cleansing shampoo. A keratolytic shampoo containing salicylic acid, and/or cleansing shampoo of preference can be used pre- and post-tar shampoo application. Unfortunately, many tar shampoos can stain or discolor gray or white hair a disagreeable yellow or greenish-yellow. Some tar shampoos, such as Ionil T®

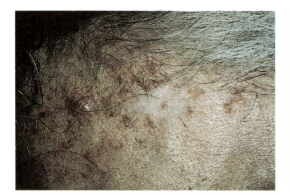

Figure 13 Scarring alopecia (erosive pustular dermatosis) in elderly female

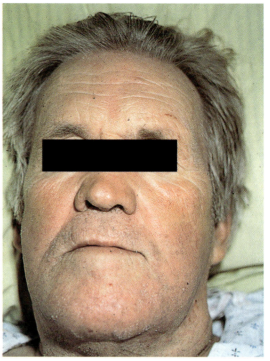

Figure 14 Seborrheic dermatitis in male with involvement of hairline, eyebrows, nasolabial folds and beard areas

(Owen/Galderma), have been especially formulated to avoid this undesirable side-effect. Zinc pyrithione, selenium sulfide, sulfur and salicylic acid shampoos are antimitotic. Ketoconazole, selenium sulfide and zinc pyrithione can reduce *P. ovale* colonization[95–98]. All shampoos should be left on for the recommended time interval. A corticosteroid solution or spray may be applied to the scalp following shampooing. There have been reports of topical and oral ketoconazole and terbinafine in the treatment of seborrheic dermatitis. Rotation of shampoos to prevent tachyphylaxis is important. The continued use of shampoos on a rotational basis should be implemented for maintenance therapy. All other grooming aids, such as conditioner, gels, mousses and hair sprays may be used concomitantly. Hair dyes and permanent waving procedures are not contraindicated.

SCALP PSORIASIS

The scalp is a site of predilection for psoriasis and is affected in 50% of patients with this condition[99]. Runne and colleagues noted that scalp involvement was the inaugural event in 66% of their patients, and in 36% the scalp was the only site involved[100]. More specifically, the preferred sites can be similar to those favored by seborrheic dermatitis, that is the retroauricular, external auditory canal and eyebrows. Figure 15 shows plaques in the retroauricular and external auditory canal. Plaques may extend well beyond the hairline, but the edges, in general, remain very sharply delineated (Figure 16). The psoriatic scale is thick and 'silvery' with better defined plaques compared with seborrheic dermatitis. The degree of inflammation also tends to be greater. Itching and scaling are the most distressing symptoms[101]. Excessive manipulation of the plaques from scratching or sharp-edged combs may provoke worsening psoriasis, a phenomenon called Knoebnerization. The constant attention required to treat psoriasis can be frustrating, and compliance may prove difficult for the elderly patient.

Hair loss may be associated with acute and chronic psoriasis. The erythrodermic form may be associated with telogen effluvium because of systemic side-effects. The hair shafts overlying psoriatic plaques often appear dry and lusterless and break easily[102].

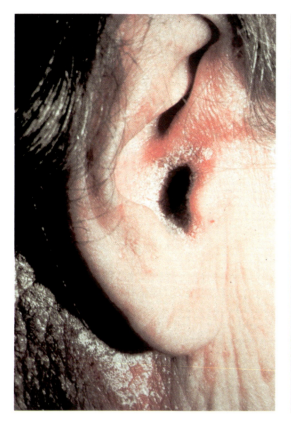

Figure 15 Psoriatic plaques in retroauricular region and external auditory canal

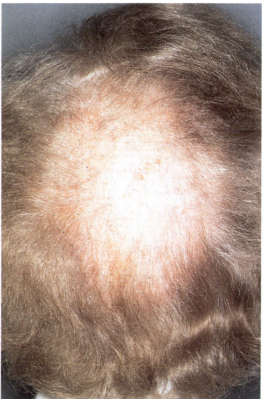

Figure 17 Scarring alopecia resulting in decreased hair density in long-standing psoriasis

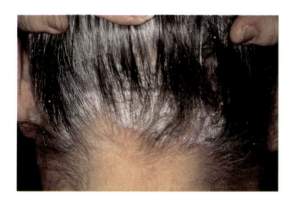

Figure 16 Thick psoriatic plaques in occipital scalp with extension on to posterior neck

Tufts or clumps of hair may be lost as the adherent scale is removed[100]. There is an anagen to telogen shift in hairs within the plaques with resultant increased shedding of telogen hairs[102,103] and reduced hair density. Runne and colleagues reported on hair loss in 47 patients and found telogen counts increased by up to 25–86%[100]. Hair loss was reported as acute in 51%, chronic in 36% and chronic-recurrent in 13%. Alopecia was patchy (75%) or diffuse (25%). With control after therapy, complete regrowth was noted in all but five patients, who showed residual thinning or scarring. Wright and Messenger have described scarring in long-standing scalp psoriasis (Figure 17)[104].

Etiology

The thickened scales are a result of proliferation of the keratinocytes, which show an increased labeling index. The external root sheath may share this phenomenon, but not the hair bulb, so hair growth rate is normal.

Activated T cells, interacting with antigen presenting cells in the dermis and epidermis, play an integral role in the pathogenesis of psoriasis. Once activated, T cells release cytokines which induce hyperproliferation of keratinocytes and further stimulation of T cells.

Treatment

Consistent adherence to a treatment regimen is necessary to control scalp psoriasis[105]. As in seborrheic dermatitis, treatment consists of removal of the scale and medicating the underlying skin. Some older individuals can manage scalp psoriasis independently. Others need help with the application of medication and shampooing. The presence of hair complicates treatment. Removal of scale is the first step. Hydration of the scalp by shampooing, soaking the scalp, or wrapping with hot towels will help to improve the effectiveness of medications. Several means may be helpful in loosening the scales. Oils (vegetable oils) with or without a corticosteroid may be left on overnight with occlusion and shampooed out the following morning using a rotation of medicated shampoos (discussed in the previous section). One such oil and corticosteroid product contains peanut oil and fluocinolone 0.01%, another contains phenol and saline. Keratolytic and antimitotic agents such as oils containing tars aid in loosening the adherent scales. After daily shampooing, corticosteroids in the form of sprays and short-term high-potency[106,107] or long-term mid-strength topical solutions can safely be used without scalp atrophy[108]. A series of Grenz ray treatments may be helpful in the acute phase[109]. A Grenz ray is a soft X-ray, intermediate between ultraviolet light and conventional X-rays, capable of by-passing hair to penetrate the scalp to a depth of approximately 4 mm. Application of UV light with a special combing device may be useful and suitable for home use[110].

Calcipotriol is effective in treating the hyperproliferation of psoriasis by its potent growth inhibiting effects and is manufactured in a solution for scalp application[111]. By performing serial hair plucks, Kuijpers and colleagues studied the effects of calcipotriol on the anagen : telogen ratio in psoriatic plaques and found them unchanged after six weeks[103]. Calcipotriol may be used in conjunction with topical corticosteroids, either sequentially or in pulse fashion. Salicylic acid reduces the potency of calcipotriol therefore they should not be combined together. Tazarotene gel, 0.05% and 0.1%, is a topical retinoid compound which can be useful for glabrous skin lesions around the hairline. Combination with topical steroids can reduce the irritancy potential of this compound. Anthralin, 0.25% and 0.1%, comes in a scalp preparation and may be used with short contact therapy, applied for 10–20 minutes, increasing duration as tolerated. All topical preparations have more potential to cause irritation on the scalp and should be applied with caution because of the occlusive effect that hair produces. Oral diflucan and itraconazole have been helpful in severe cases[112]. Oral treatment with methotrexate, acitretin and cyclosporin is rarely indicated for use in the treatment of scalp psoriasis unless patients have severe psoriasis elsewhere. This is especially true in the geriatric population, who may be more at risk for side-effects. Secondary infections should be treated with appropriate antibiotics.

Histology

There are several features of early involvement of the skin and follicles with follicular plugging, enlargement of the follicular ostium, follicular parakeratosis, mild acanthosis and irregular hyperkeratosis. The outer root sheath and hair matrix are not affected. Other common findings include sebaceous gland atrophy, reduction of follicular size and decrease in hair shaft diameter[113]. Scarring can occur in severe psoriasis caused by inflammatory destruction of the follicle[104].

DERMATOMYOSITIS

Dermatomyositis is a rare, inflammatory myopathy manifested by progressive proximal muscle weakness, either isolated (polymyositis) or in combination with a constellation of skin manifestations: erythema of the forearms and upper back, painful scaly erythematous papules over the joints (Grotron's papules), edema and heliotrope discoloration on the upper eyelids, and scalp involvement characterized by atrophic, scaly, erythematous plaques mimicking psoriasis or seborrheic dermatitis. It can be classified as adult idiopathic, juvenile, amyopathic as well as being associated with internal malignancy[114]. There are two peaks of age of onset – childhood and over forty, though peak incidence is in the fifth and sixth decades.

In one study of 17 consecutive patients, 14 had scalp involvement at the time of diagnosis, 6 of whom had hair loss[115]. McDonald and Smith report on scalp scaling and dermatomyositis in the pediatric population as well[116]. Various reports indicate a 12–34% association with internal malignancies, with the majority of these individuals over 40 years old[114,115,117–120]. The source of the malignancies are gastrointestinal, breast, ovarian, lung and melanoma. In the literature from Japan[117] and Singapore[119], nasopharyngeal carcinoma predominates; 31% of malignancies addressed in Singapore originated in the nasopharynx[119]. Wong reported that 74% of malignancies in 23 cases in a Chinese population originated in the nasopharynx[121]. Koh and colleagues reported an older age group (mean 61.8 years) and higher percentage of associated malignancy in patients with dermatomyositis compared with polymyositis[118]. Recognition of the scalp involvement is important as it may be the presenting complaint in some patients with dermatomyositis. Early diagnosis will alert the treating physician to evaluate patients for possible associated malignancies.

INFECTIOUS SCALP DISORDERS

Only two infectious scalp disorders will be discussed as related to the geriatric population. Tinea capitis in the elderly is unusual but increasing in incidence and should be considered in the differential diagnosis of inflammatory and non-inflammatory conditions of the scalp. Herpes zoster of the trigeminal distribution takes a particularly large toll in morbidity on the elderly.

TINEA CAPITIS

In North America *Trichophyton tonsurans* is becoming the most common causative agent of tinea capitis, followed by *Microsporum canis*. *Microsporum audouinii*, formerly the most common cause of tinea capitis in the United States, typically occurred in prepubertal children and cleared spontaneously in postpubertal adolescence. Tinea capitis caused by *Trichophyton tonsurans* may persist into adulthood and may affect multiple generations. In Europe *Trichophyton violaceum* and *Microsporum canis* have replaced *Trichophyton schoenleinii* as the most frequent etiologic agents.

Tinea capitis is becoming more prevalent in all age groups and should be excluded in older patients with unusual or unresponsive scalp conditions. Any dermatophyte causing disease in children can cause tinea capitis in adults[122]. When present, lesions are variable and often atypical. It is more common in adult and elderly women than men, for unexplained reasons[122–124]. Moberg in 1984 reported on two elderly women with tinea capitis caused by *Trichophyton tonsurans*[125]. One had scalp scaling mimicking seborrheic dermatitis. The other had lesions mimicking discoid lupus erythematosus. Connerly and Greer reported an 89-year-old black female with generalized folliculitis that proved to be tinea capitis caused by *Trichophyton tonsurans*[126] and Schwinn and co-workers reported two cases of tinea capitis caused by *Trichophyton rubrum*, generally considered an unusual etiological organism[127].

The presence of asymptomatic carriers is becoming increasingly important. One survey demonstrated that 30% of adults exposed to a child infected with *T. tonsurans* were colonized[128]. In another study, it was estimated that half of the children infected with

T. tonsurans had at least one adult contact who was culture positive[129]. Older individuals who live with or have frequent contact with infected children, especially in crowded conditions, should be considered at risk.

Clinical presentation

As discussed above, the asymptomatic carrier may have little evidence of infection other than non-inflammatory scaling. The signs of infection may be variable and unusual. Diffuse or patchy alopecia, folliculitis, pustules or crusting may be seen in those with more inflammatory infections.

Diagnosis

Direct microscopic examination of infected hairs and/or scales which have been prepared with 25% KOH solution will show the hyphal elements in scales or the spores in infected hairs. The spores may be external to the hair shaft as in *Microsporum canis* (ectothrix infection) or inside the hair shaft itself as in *Trichophyton tonsurans* (endothrix infection). Diagnosis can be confirmed by culture on an appropriate mycology medium.

Treatment

Oral therapy is generally necessary for treatment of tinea capitis. Griseofulvin has been the standard therapy for decades. Long-term treatment is necessary to achieve a cure and can potentially be a deterrent to therapy, especially in the elderly patient for whom compliance may be difficult. Newer oral agents have shown promise in treatment. The azole antifungals fluconazole and itraconazole and the allylamine antifungal terbinafine have all been studied in comparative trials and may be appropriate for second-line therapy[130]. Adjunctive therapy with 2% ketoconazole or 2.5% selenium sulfide shampoo, allowed to remain on the scalp for five minutes three times weekly, should be added to oral therapy to aid in the eradication of infection[131].

HERPES ZOSTER

The herpes zoster virus can involve the scalp when the ophthalmic branch of the trigeminal nerve becomes involved. Diagnosis can be made clinically and by Tzank smear. It presents as grouped vesicles along a dermatomal distribution. The vesicles can evolve into crusts and occasionally ulcerations (Figure 18). Pain may be severe. It is estimated that 300 000 new cases of herpes zoster are seen in the United States each year[132]. Several factors influence the incidence, with increasing age being the most consistent[132,133]. Post-herpetic neuralgia is the number one cause of intractable, debilitating pain in the elderly and is the leading cause of suicide in chronic pain patients over the age of 70 years[132].

The onset is often preceded by a prodrome consisting of pain, itching and paresthesias. Prodromal pain, pain during acute phase infection and post-herpetic neuralgia are more commonly experienced by patients over 50 years old. Comorbidity symptoms such as insomnia are common in the elderly[134]. Post-herpetic neuralgia is a serious consequence of herpes zoster and occurs more commonly and lasts longer in patients over 60 years old[133,135]. It is often severe and refractory to treatment. More than 50% of patients with herpes zoster over 60 years of age will develop post-herpetic neuralgia which may persist for months or even years[133]. It is more common in those with trigeminal involvement. Higa and colleagues found that the extent of the involvement of the skin correlates with the duration of post-herpetic pain in all age groups[135]. However, patients over 60 years old had more extensive lesions. Involvement of the cornea is considered a medical emergency causing keratoconjunctivitis, uveitis and ocular motor paralysis[136]. Hair loss and eventual scarring may occur in areas of ulceration.

Treatment

Acute herpes zoster antiviral treatment has changed in recent years. The efficacy of

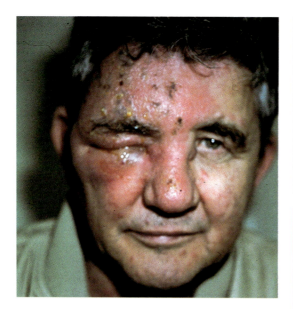

Figure 18 Herpes zoster involving ophthalmic branch of trigeminal nerve

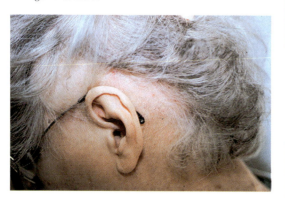

Figure 19 Late-onset alopecia areata with ophiasis distribution

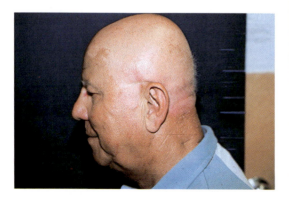

Figure 20 Late onset alopecia areata universalis with vitiligo

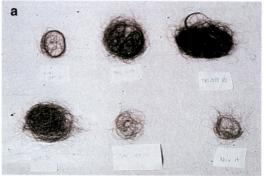

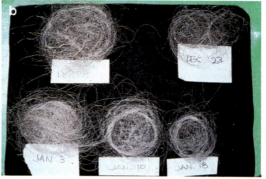

Figure 21 Pigmented hairs are sometimes shed preferentially in alopecia areata. In this patient, only pigmented hairs were shed initially, followed by shedding of unpigmented hairs 4 months later

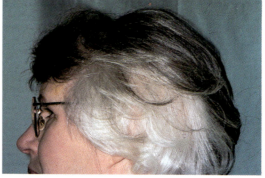

Figure 22 Permanent white hair regrowth in areas of alopecia areata

valacyclovir, the prodrug of acyclovir, and that of famciclovir[137], the prodrug of penciclovir, have been documented in large clinical trials[138,139]. Both drugs are effective on herpes zoster-associated pain and in shortening the course of the disease. Development of resistance against acyclovir and the nucleoside analogs in the treatment of immunocompetent individuals has not become a problem. Famciclovir and valacyclovir allow for less frequent daily dosing and higher concentrations of serum drug concentration. Initiation of therapy as soon as possible is advised. Famciclovir, 500 mg t.i.d. for one week, and valacyclovir, 1 g t.i.d. for one week are the recommended dosages. Prednisone in cases of trigeminal involvement has been shown to be beneficial[140,141].

Post-herpetic pain presents a therapeutic challenge. Tricyclic antidepressants, gabapentin[142] and sympathetic nerve blocks with xylocaine, bupivacaine and dexamethasone[143] have all been reported with some successes. Chiarello[144] reports administering corticosteroids, lidocaine and epinephrine in a tumescent technique. Administration in the facial area must be performed cautiously using 100–250 ml of fluid, injecting superficially and slowly, allowing percolation into the deeper tissues. Iontophoresis with lidocaine and methylprednisolone[145] and antiviral drugs[146] has shown long-term efficacy in 60–90% of patients treated.

ALOPECIA AREATA

Alopecia areata is an inflammatory, non-scarring form of hair loss characterized by round or oval patches of complete hair loss. Any hair-bearing area can be affected. The loss can progress to loss of all scalp hair (alopecia totalis) or complete loss of all hair on the body (alopecia universalis). There are several distinctive forms affecting between 0.1% and 0.2% of the population[147]. Twelve per cent of cases initially present over the age of 50 years. In these patients it may present with any form seen in other age groups: patchy, ophiasis, reverse ophiasis, reticulate, diffuse, totalis and universalis. In both cases, seen in Figures 19 and 20, this was the patient's first episode of alopecia areata. The geriatric population is more likely to present with the expression of other autoimmune diseases, if genetically susceptible. It is recognized that alopecia areata may preferentially attack pigmented hairs and may spare white hair. Patients with significant numbers of gray or white hairs may shed pigmented hairs only. Figure 21 (a & b) shows sequential hair loss in one individual over some four months; pigmented hairs were lost before unpigmented ones. The patient was left entirely white haired. This may explain the phenomenon of apparent rapid graying of hair. When hair regrows, it may grow as white hair only, initially or permanently (Figure 22). Although alopecia areata tends to be more severe when presenting in younger age groups, it can be extensive and aggressive even in geriatric patients with a first episode.

Etiology

The etiology of alopecia areata is unknown, although an autoimmune pathogenesis has been frequently proposed. Support for this hypothesis is provided by the increased association with other autoimmune disorders such as hyper- and hypothyroid disorders, vitiligo, lupus erythematosus, discoid lupus erythematosus, rheumatoid arthritis, premature ovarian failure, pernicious anemia and ulcerative colitis. There is a high prevalence of auto-antibodies against thyroid, gastric parietal cells, nuclear constituents and rheumatoid factors[148,149]. Forty per cent of patients with alopecia areata have an atopic diasthesis including allergic rhinitis, asthma or atopic dermatitis[150] (see Figure 4). Between 10% and 27% of patients have a family history of alopecia areata[151].

Melanocytes are suspected to be one target of the immune attack. It is well known that pigmented hairs are affected preferentially and that the senile white or gray hairs may be spared. There is also an increased association with vitiligo. Tobin and colleagues found increased numbers of bizarre melanosomes in affected melanocytes, indicating the active involvement of hair bulb melanocytes[152]. Messenger and Bleehan examined the regrowing white hairs in seven patients, finding that the number of melanocytes and melanization were less than in normal pigmented follicles, and suggested that pigmentary mechanisms in the hair bulb, especially in senile white hairs, are of primary importance in the pathogenesis[153].

Treatment

Treatment can be divided into immunomodulators (oral, intralesional, intramuscular corticosteroids, cyclosporin, ultraviolet light with or without PUVA), immunostimulants (for example topical squaric acid dibutyl ester (SADBE), diphenylcyclopropenone (DPCP) and anthralin) and non-specific hair follicle growth promoters (minoxidil). Corticosteroids require careful monitoring in the geriatric population, whether administered by the oral, intralesional or intramuscular routes, because of the potential for serious side-effects. These include causing or potentiating cataracts, glaucoma, hypertension, hyperglycemia and osteoporosis.

In the author's experience, older individuals are more likely to be accepting of hair loss and less willing to try various treatments for extensive alopecia areata, settling for a nicely styled hairpiece. Contact sensitization with SADBE or DPCP may by attempted, although older individuals may be more difficult to sensitize to these chemicals. Patient preference should always be taken into account. The less aggressive patchy forms can be addressed with long-term topical or intralesional corticosteroids or anthralin cream or 5% topical minoxidil. Interested readers are referred for further reading to Alopecia Areata Update[154].

References

1. Freedman TG. Social and cultural dimensions of hair loss in women treated for breast cancer. *Cancer Nurs* 1994;17:334–41
2. Cash TF, Price VH, Savin RC. Psychological effects of androgenetic alopecia on women: comparisons with balding men and with female control subjects. *J Am Acad Dermatol* 1993;29:568–75
3. Pickard-Holley S. The symptom experience of alopecia. *Semin Oncol Nurs* 1995;11:235–8
4. Dawber R, Van-Neste D. Hair Color. In *Hair and Scalp Disorders*. London: Martin Dunitz and Philadelphia: JB Lippincott, 1995:236–8
5. Bartosova L, Strava Z, Jorda V. Clinical trichology. *Curr Probl Dermatol* 1984;12:163–6
6. Fitzpatrick T, Szabo G, Mitchell R. Age changes in the human melanocyte system. In Montagna W, ed. *Advances in Biology of the Skin*, Vol 6. Oxford: Pergamon Press, 1965:35–60
7. Fitzpatrick TB, Brunet P, Kubita A. The nature of hair pigment. In Montagna W, Ellis RA, eds. *The Biology of Hair Growth*. New York: Academic Press, 1958:255–303
8. Hsieh SD, Yamamot R, Saito K, *et al.* Amyloidosis presented with whitening and loss of hair which improved after dimethyl sulfoxide (DMSO) treatment. *Jpn J Med* 1987;26:393–5
9. Sato S, Kubita A, Jimbow K. Electron microscopic studies of dendritic cells in the human gray and white hair matrix during anagen. In McGovern V, Russell P, eds. *Pigment Cell*, Vol 1. Basel: Karger, 1987:20–7
10. Noppakun N, Swasdikul D. Reversible hyperpigmentation of skin and nails with white hair due to vitamin B12 deficiency. *Arch Dermatol* 1986;122:896–9
11. Messenger A. The control of hair growth and pigmentation. In Olsen EA, ed. *Disorders of Hair Growth; Diagnosis and Treatment*. New York: McGraw-Hill, 1994:54–5
12. Verbov J. Erosive candidiasis of the scalp, followed by reappearance of black hair after 40 years. *Br J Dermatol* 1981;105:595–8
13. Comaish S. White scalp hairs turning black – an unusual reversal of the aging process. *Br J Dermatol* 1972;86:513–14
14. Schnohr P, Lange P, Nyboe J, *et al.* Gray hair, baldness, and wrinkles in relation to myocardial infarction, the Copenhagen City Heart Study. *Am Heart J* 1995;130:1003–10
15. Glasser M. Is early onset of gray hair a risk factor? *Med Hypothesis* 1991;36:404–11
16. Cotsarelis G, Sun TT, Lavker RM. Label-retaining cells reside in the bulge area of

pilosebaceous unit: implications for follicular stem cells, hair cycle and skin. *Cell* 1990;61: 1329–37

17. Abell E. Embryology and anatomy of the hair follicle. In Olsen EA, ed. *Disorders of Hair Growth: Diagnosis and Treatment*. New York: McGraw-Hill, 1994:7

18. Kligman A. The comparative histopathology of male-pattern baldness and senescent baldness. *Clin Dermatol* 1988;6:108–18

19. Pinkus H. Alopecia. Clinicopathologic correlations. *Int J Dermatol* 1980;19:245–53

20. Rebora A. Telogen effluvium. *Dermatology* 1997;195:209–12

21. Headington JT. Telogen effluvium. New concepts and review. *Arch Dermatol* 1993;129: 356–63

22. Skelton JB. Postpartum alopecia. *Am J Obstet Gynecol* 1966;95:125–9

23. Schiff BL, Pawtucket RI, Kern AB. Study of postpartum alopecia. *Arch Dermatol* 1963;87: 609–11

24. Hard S. Non anemic iron deficiency as etiologic factor in diffuse loss of hair in the scalp of women. *Acta Derm Venereol* 1965;43: 562–9

25. Bernstein GM, Crollick JS, Hassett JM. Postfebrile telogen effluvium in critically ill patients. *Crit Care Med* 1988;16:98–9

26. Broden MB. Drug-related alopecia. *Dermatol Clin* 1987;5:571–9

27. Jordan VE. Protein status of the elderly as measured by dietary intake, hair tissue and serum albumin. *Am J Clin Nutr* 1976;29:522–8

28. Church RE. Hypothyroid hair loss. *Br J Dermatol* 1965;77:661–2

29. Freinkel RK, Freinkel N. Hair growth and alopecia and hypothyroidism. *Arch Dermatol* 1972;106:349–52

30. Comaish JS. The thyroid and hair growth. *Semin Dermatol* 1985;4:4–8

31. Kay RG, Tasman Jones C. Acute zinc deficiency in man during intravenous alimentation. *Aust NZ J Surg* 1975;45:325–30

32. Tucker SB, Schroeter AL, Brown PW, McCall JT. Acquired zinc deficiency. *J Am Med Assoc* 1976;235:2399–402

33. Weismann K, Wadskov S, Mikkelsen HI, *et al.* Acquired zinc deficiency dermatosis in man. *Arch Dermatol* 1978;114:1509–11

34. Tosti A, Mesciali C, Peroccini BM, *et al.* Drug induced hair loss and hair growth. Incidence, management and avoidance. *Drug Saf* 1994; 10:310–17

35. Whiting DA. Chronic telogen effluvium. *Dermatol Clin* 1996;14:723–31

36. Rushton DH, Ramsay ID. The importance of adequate serum ferritin levels during oral cyproterone acetate and ethinyl oestradiol

treatment on diffuse androgen-dependent alopecia in women. *Clin Endocrinol* 1992;36: 421–7

37. Graeber CW, Lapkin RA. Metoprolol and alopecia. *Cutis* 1981;28:633–4

38. Fraunfelder FT, Meyer SM, Menacker SJ. Alopecia possibly secondary to topical ophthalmic β-blockers. *J Am Med Assoc* 1990; 263:1493–4

39. Martin CM, Southwick EG, Maibach HI. Propranolol-induced alopecia. *Am Heart J* 1973; 86:236–7

40. Miki Y. Alopecia from heparin. *Med J Osaka Univ* 1960;11:315–23

41. Robinson MH, Jones HC, Durrant KD. Effectiveness of scalp cooling in reducing alopecia caused by epirubicin treatment of advanced breast cancer. *Cancer Treat Rep* 1987;71:913–14

42. Ron IG, Kalmus Y, Kalmus Z, *et al.* Scalp cooling in the prevention of alopecia in patients receiving depilating chemotherapy. *Support Care Cancer* 1997;5:136–8

43. Tollenaar RA, Liefers GF, Repelaer-va-Driel OJ, Van-de-Velde CJ. Scalp cooling has no place in adjuvant chemotherapy for breast cancer. *Eur J Cancer* 1994;30A:1448–53

44. Ebling FJ. The biology of hair. *Dermatol Clin* 1987;5:467–81

45. Courtois M, Loussouarn G, Hourseau C, Grollier JF. Ageing and hair cycles. *Br J Dermatol* 1995;132:86–93

46. Roberts JL. Androgenetic alopecia in men and women: an overview of cause and treatment. *Dermatol Nurs* 1997;9:379–86

47. Hamilton JB, Patterned loss of hair in man: types and incidence. *Ann NY Acad Sci* 1951; 53:708–28

48. Norwood OT. Male pattern baldness: classification and incidence. *South Med J* 1975; 68:1359–65

49. Olsen EA. Androgenetic alopecia. In Olsen EA, ed. *Disorders of Hair Growth, Diagnosis and Treatment*. New York: McGraw-Hill, 1994: 257–83

50. Venning VA, Dawber RPR. Patterned androgenetic alopecia in women. *J Am Acad Dermatol* 1988;18:1073–7

51. Imperato-McGinley J, Guerrero L, Gautier R, Peterson RE. Steroid 5α reductase deficiency in man: an inherited form of male pseudohermaphroditism. *Science* 1974;186: 1213–15

52. Sawaya ME, Price VH. Different levels of 5-alpha reductase types I and II, aromatase, and androgen receptors in hair follicles of women and men with androgenetic alopecia. *J Invest Dermatol* 1997;109:296–300

53. Van Neste D, Fuh V, Sanchez-Pedreno P, *et al.* Finasteride in the treatment of men

with androgenetic alopecia using a photo-trichogram technique. *Society for Investigative Dermatology*, Chicago, IL, May 1999

54. Kaufman KD, Olsen EA, Whiting DA, *et al.* Finasteride in the treatment of men with androgenetic alopecia. *J Am Acad Dermatol* 1998;39:578–89

55. Roberts JL, Hordinsky M, Olsen E, *et al.* The effects of finasteride on post-menopausal women with androgenetic alopecia. *Hair Workshop (abstract)*; Brussels, Belgium, May 2–3, 1998:16

56. Uno H, Cappas A, Brigham P. Action of topical minoxidil in the bald stump-tailed macaque. *J Am Acad Dermatol* 1987;16:657–68

57. Headington JT. Hair follicle biology and topical minoxidil: possible mechanism of action. *Dermatologica* 1987;175(Suppl 2):19–22

58. Roberts JL. Androgenetic alopecia: treatment results with topical minoxidil. *J Am Acad Dermatol* 1987;1:705–10

59. Lesko SM, Rosenberg L, Shapiro S. A case-control study of baldness in relation to myocardial infarction in men. *J Am Med Assoc* 1993;269:998–1003

60. Ford ES, Frudman DS, Byers T. Baldness and ischemic heart disease in a national sample of men. Comment in: *Am J Epidemiol* 1997;145:670–1

61. Herrera R, D'Agostino RB, Girstman BB, *et al.* Baldness and coronary heart disease in men from the Framingham study. *Am J Epidemiol* 1995;142:828–33

62. Trevisan M, *et al.* Baldness and coronary heart disease risk factors. *J Clin Epidemiol* 1993;46:1213–18

63. Halim MM, Meyrick G, Jeans WD, *et al.* Myocardial infarction, androgen and the skin. *Br J Dermatol* 1978;98:63–8

64. Cooke NT. Male pattern alopecia and coronary heart disease in men. *Br J Dermatol* 1979;101:455–8

65. Maguire HC Jr, Kligman AM. The histopathology of common male baldness. *Excerpta Medica Found* 1962;55:1438–9

66. Young JW, Conte ET, Leavitt ML, *et al.* Cutaneous immunopathology of androgenetic alopecia. *J Am Osteopathic Assoc* 1991;91:765–71

67. Lattanand A, Johnson WC. Male pattern alopecia: a histopathologic and histochemical study. *J Cutan Pathol* 1975;2:58–70

68. Jaworsky C, Kligman AM, Murphy GF. Characterization of inflammatory infiltrates in male pattern alopecia: implications for pathogenesis. *Br J Dermatol* 1992;127:239–46

69. Smith WB, Grabski WJ, McCollough ML, Davis TL. Immunofluorescence findings in lichen planopilaris. A contrasting experience (letter). *Arch Dermatol* 1992;128:1405–6

70. Ioannides D, Bystryn JC. Immunofluorescence abnormalities in lichen planopilaris. *Arch Dermatol* 1992;128:214–16

71. Elston DM, Bergfeld WF. Cicatricial alopecia (and other causes of permanent alopecia). In Olsen EA, ed. *Disorders of Hair Growth: Diagnosis and Treatment.* New York: McGraw-Hill, 1994:285–313

72. Kossard S. Postmenopausal frontal fibrosing alopecia. Scarring in pattern distribution. *Arch Dermatol* 1994;130:770–4

73. Feldmann R, Harmes M, Saurat JH. Postmenopausal frontal fibrosing alopecia. *Hautarzt* 1996;47:533–6

74. Lee WS, Hwang SM, Ahan SK. Frontal fibrosing alopecia in a postmenopausal woman. *Cutis* 1997;60:299–300

75. Trueb RM, Torricelli R. Lichen planopilaris simulating frontal fibrosing alopecia. *Hautarzt* 1998;49:388–91

76. Kossard S, Lee MS, Wilkinson B. Postmenopausal frontal fibrosing alopecia: a frontal variant of lichen planopilaris. *J Am Acad Dermatol* 1997;36:59–66

77. Mehregan DA, Van Hale HM, Muller SA. Lichen planopilaris: clinical and pathological study of forty-five patients. *J Am Acad Dermatol* 1992;27:935–42

78. Elston DM, McCollough ML, Angeloni VL. Vertical and transverse sections of alopecia biopsy specimens: combining the two to maximize diagnostic yield. *J Am Acad Dermatol* 1995;32:454–7

79. Pye RJ, Peachey RD, Burton JL. Erosive pustular dermatosis of the scalp. *Br J Dermatol* 1979;100:559–66

80. Caputo R, Veraldi S. Erosive pustular dermatosis of the scalp. *J Am Acad Dermatol* 1993;28:96–8

81. Watanbe S, Takizawa K, Hashimoto N, Ishibashi Y. Pustular dermatosis of the scalp associated with autoimmune diseases. *J Dermatol* 1989;16:383–7

82. Noe C, Grob JJ, Choux R, Bonerandi JJ. Erosive pustolosis of the scalp. A spongiform pustular dermatosis? *Ann Dermatol Venereol* 1993;120:693–5

83. Ena P, Lissia M, Doneduu GM, Campus GV. Erosive pustular dermatosis of the scalp in skin grafts: report of three cases. *Dermatology* 1997;194:80–4

84. Wollenberg A, Heckmann M, Braun-Falco O. Erosive pustular dermatosis of the scalp after zoster opthalmicus and trauma. *Hautarzt* 1992;43:576–9

85. Jacyk WK. Pustular dermatosis of the scalp. *Br J Dermatol* 1988;118:441–4

86. Pye RJ, Peachey RD, Burton JL. Erosive pustular dermatosis of the scalp. *Br J Dermatol* 1979; 100:559–66

87. Sperling LC, Sau P. The follicular degeneration syndrome in black patients. 'Hot comb alopecia' revisited and revised. *Arch Dermatol* 1992;128:68–74

88. Sperling LC, Skelton HG, Smith KJ, *et al*. Follicular degeneration syndrome in men. *Arch Dermatol* 1994;130:763–9

89. Tarkowski E, Jensen C, Ekholm S, *et al*. Localization of the brain lesions affects the laterlization of T-lymphocyte dependent cutaneous inflammation. Evidence for immunoregulatory role of the right frontal cortex-putamen region. *Scand J Immunol* 1998;47:30–6

90. Martignoni E, Godi, Pacchetti C, *et al*. Is seborrhea a sign of autonomic impairment in Parkinson's disease? *J Neural Transm* 1997; 104:1295–304

91. Binder RL, Jonelis FJ, Seborrheic dermatitis in neuroleptic-induced Parkinsonism. *Arch Dermatol* 1983;119:473–5

92. Flint A. The skin in Parkinson's disease. *Prim Care* 1977;4:475–80

93. Neuber K, Kroger S, Grusek E, *et al*. Effects of *Pityrosporum ovale* on proliferation, immunoglobulin (IgA, G, M) synthesis and cytokine (IL-2, II-10, IFN gamma) production of peripheral blood mononuclear cells from patients with seborrheic dermatitis. *Arch Dermatol Res* 1996;288:532–6

94. Bergbrant IM. Seborrhoeic dermatitis and *Pityrosporum* yeasts. *Curr Top Med Mycol* 1995; 6:95–112

95. Peter RU, Richarz-Barthauer U. Successful treatment and prophylaxis of scalp seborrheic dermatitis and dandruff with 2% ketoconazole shampoo. *Br J Dermatol* 1995; 132:441–5

96. Nenoff P, Huastein UF, Munzberger C. *In vitro* activity of lithium succinate against. *Malassezia furfur. Dermatology* 1995;190:48–50

97. Danby FW, Maddin WS, Margesson J, Rosenthal D. A randomized, placebo-controlled trial of ketoconazole as shampoo versus selenium 2.5% shampoo in the treatment of moderate to severe dandruff. *J Am Acad Dermatol* 1993;29:1008–12

98. Faergemann J. *Pityrosporum* infections. *J Am Acad Dermatol* 1994;31:S18–20

99. Farber EM, Nall L. Natural history and treatment of scalp psoriasis. *Cutis* 1992;49: 396–400

100. Runne U, Kroneisen-Wiersma P. Psoriatic alopecia; acute and chronic hair loss in 47 patients with scalp psoriasis [published

101. van-de-Kerhof PC, de-Hoop D, de-Korte J, Kuipers MV. Scalp psoriasis, clinical presentations and therapeutic management. *Dermatology*1998;197:326–34

102. Stanimirovic A, Skerlev M, Stipic T, *et al*. Has psoriasis its own characteristic trichogram? *J Dermatol Sci* 1998;17:156–9

103. Kuijpers AL, van-Baar HM, van-Gasselt MW, van-de-Kerkhof PC. The hair root pattern after calcipotriol treatment for scalp psoriasis. *Acta Derm Venereol* 1995;75:388–90

104. Wright AL, Messenger AG. Scarring alopecia in psoriasis. *Acta Derm Venereol* 1990;70:156–9

105. Boyd AS. Scalp psoriasis. *Am Fam Physician* 1988;38:163–70

106. Olsen EA, Cram DL, Ellis CN, *et al*. A double-blind, vehicle-controlled study of clobetasol propionate 0.05% (Temovate) scalp application in the treatment of moderate to severe scalp psoriasis. *J Am Acad Dermatol* 1991; 24:443–7

107. Katz HI, Lindholm JS, Weiss JS, *et al*. Efficacy and safety of twice-daily augmented betamethasone dipropionate lotion versus clobetasol propionate solution in patients with moderate-to-severe scalp psoriasis. *Clin Ther* 1995;17:390–401

108. Prakash A, Benfield P. Topical mometasone. A review of its pharmacological properties and therapeutic use in the treatment of dermatological disorders. *Drugs* 1998;55: 145–63

109. Johannesson A, Lindelof B. Additional effect of Grenz rays on psoriasis lesions of the scalp treated with topical corticosteroids. *Dermatologica* 1987;175:290–2

110. Caccialanza M, Piccinno R, Cappio F, *et al*. Phototherapy of psoriasis of the scalp. Results in 21 patients treated with a special portable ultraviolet rays lamp. *G Ital Dermatol Venereol* 1989;124:LXI–LXV

111. Klaber MR, Hutchinson PE, Pedvis-Leftick A, *et al*. Comparative effects of calcipotriol solution (50 micrograms/ml) and betamethasone 17-valerate solution (1mg/ml) in the treatment of scalp psoriasis. *Br J Dermatol* 1994;131:678–83

112. Faergemann J. Treatment of sebopsoriasis with itraconazole. *Mykosen* 1985;28:612–18

113. Wilson CL, Dean D, Lane EB, *et al*. Keratinocyte differentiation in psoriatic scalp: morphology and expression of epithelial keratins. *Br J Dermatol* 1994;131:191–200

114. Maoz CR, Langevitz P, Leyneh A, *et al*. High incidence of malignancies with dermatomyositis and polymyositis: an 11-year analysis.

erratum appears in *Dermatology* 1993; 187:232]. *Dermatology* 1992;185(2):82–7

Seminars in Arthritis and Rheumatism 1998; 27:319–24

115. Kasteler JS, Callen JP. Scalp involvement in dermatomyositis. Often overlooked or misdiagnosed. *J Am Med Assoc* 1994;272:1939–41

116. McDonald LL, Smith ML. Diagnostic dilemmas in pediatric/adolescent dermatology: scaly scalp. *J Pediatr Health Care* 1998;12:80–4

117. Hatada T, Aoki I, Ikeda H, *et al.* Dermatomyositis and malignancy: case report and review of the Japanese literature. *Tumori* 1996;82:273–5

118. Koh ET, Seow-Ong B, Ratnyopal P, *et al.* Adult onset polymyositis/dermatomyositis: clinical and laboratory features in 75 patients. *Ann Rheum Dis* 1993;52:857–61

119. Peng JC, Sheen TS, Hsu MM. Nasopharyngeal carcinoma dermatomyositis: analysis of 12 cases. *Arch Otolaryngol Head Neck Surg* 1995;121:1298–301

120. Davis MD, Ahmed I. Ovarian malignancy in patients with dermatomyositis and polymyositis: a retrospective analysis of 14 cases. *J Am Acad Dermatol* 1997;37:730–3

121. Wong KO. Dermatomyositis: a clinical investigation of twenty-three cases in Hong Kong. *Br J Dermatol* 1969;81:544–7

122. Teragni L, Lasagni A, Oreoni A. Tinea capitis in adults. *Mycoses* 1989;32:482–6

123. Pursley TV, Raimer SS. Tinea capitis in the elderly. *Int J Dermatol* 1980;19:220

124. Ridely CM. Tinea capitis in an elderly woman. *Clin Exp Dermatol* 1979;4:247–9

125. Moberg S. Tinea capitis in the elderly. A report on two cases caused by *Trichophyton tonsurans*. *Dermatologica* 1984;169:36–40

126. Conerly SL, Greer DL. Tinea capitis in adults over fifty years of age. *Cutis* 1988;41: 251–2

127. Schwinn A, Ebert J, Brocker EB. Frequency of *Trichophyton rubrum* in tinea capitis. *Mycoses* 1995;38:1–7

128. Williams JV, Honig PJ, McGinley KJ, Leyden JJ. Semiquantitative study of tinea capitis and the asymptomatic carrier state in inner-city school children. *Pediatrics* 1995;96:265–7

129. Babel DE, Baughman SA. Evaluation of the adult carrier state in juvenile tinea capitis caused by *Trichophyton tonsurans*. *J Am Acad Dermatol* 1989;21:1209–12

130. Gupta AK, Sauder DN, Shear NH. Antifungal agents: an overview. Part II. *J Am Acad Dermatol* 1994;30:911–33

131. Allen HB, Honig PJ, Leyden JJ, McGinley KJ. Selenium sulfide: adjunctive therapy for tinea capitis. *Pediatrics* 1982;69:81–3

132. Hess TM, Lutz LJ, Nauss LA, Lamer TJ. Treatment of acute herpetic neuralgia. A case report and review of the literature (see comments). *Minn Med* 1990;73:37–40

133. Gershon AA. Epidemiology and management of post herpetic neuralgia. *Semin Dermatol* 1996;15(Suppl 1):8–13

134. Goh CL, Khoo L. A retrospective study of the clinical presentation and outcome of herpes zoster in a tertiary dermatology outpatient referral clinic. *Int J Dermatol* 1997;36:667–72

135. Higa K, Mori M, Hirata K, *et al.* Severity of skin lesions of herpes zoster at the worst phase rather than age and involved region most influences the duration of acute herpes zoster pain. *Pain* 1997;69:245–53

136. Schoenlaub P, Grange F, Nasica X, Guillaume JC. Oculomotor nerve paralysis with complete ptosis in herpes zoster ophthalmicus. *Ann Dermatol Venereol* 1997;125:401–3

137. Tyring SK. Efficacy of famciclovir in the treatment of herpes zoster. *Semin Dermatol* 1996; 15(Suppl 1):27–31

138. Wutzler P. Antiviral therapy of herpes simplex and varicella zoster virus infections. *Intervirology* 1997;40:343–56

139. Erlich KS. Management of herpes simplex and varicella-zoster virus infections. *West J Med* 1997;166:211–15

140. Lycka BA. Postherpetic pain neuralgia and systemic corticosteroid therapy. *Int J Dermatol* 1990;29:523–7

141. Post BT, Philbrick JT. Do corticosteroids prevent postherpetic neuralgia? A review of the evidence. *J Am Acad Dermatol* 1988;18: 605–10

142. Rowbotham M, Harden N, Stacey B, *et al.* Gabapentin for the treatment of postherpetic neuralgia: a randomized controlled trial. *J Am Med Assoc* 1998;280:1837–42

143. Bhargava R, Bhargava S, Haldia KN, Bhargava P. Jaipur block in postherpetic neuralgia. *Int J Dermatol* 1998;37:465–8

144. Chiarello SE. Tumescent infiltration of corticosteroids, lidocaine and epinephrine into dermatomes of acute herpetic pain or posttherpetic neuralgia. *Arch Dermatol* 1998; 134:279–81

145. Ozawa A, Haruki Y, Iwashita K, *et al.* Follow-up of clinical efficacy of iontophoresis therapy for post herpetic neuralgia. *J Dermatol* 1999; 26:1–10

146. Gangarosa LP Sr, Ozawa A, Ohkido M, *et al.* Iontophoresis for enhancing penetration of dermatologic and antiviral drugs. *J Dermatol* 1995;22:865–75

147. Safavi K. Prevalence of alopecia areata in the First National Health and Nutrition Examination Survey. *Arch Dermatol* 1992;128: 702–12

148. Friedmann PS. Alopecia areata and auto-immunity. *Br J Dermatol* 1981;105:153–7

149. Schenk EA, Schneider P, Brown AC. Autoantibodies in alopecia and vitiligo. In Brown AC, Crounse RG, eds. *Hair, Trace Elements and Human Illness*. New York: Praeger, 1980:334–43

150. Young E, Bruns HM, Berrens L. Alopecia areata and atopy: a clinical study. *Dermatologica* 1984;156:306–8

151. Suader DN, Bergfeld WF, Krakauer RS. Alopecia areata: an inherited autoimmune disease. In Brown AC, Crounse RG, eds. *Hair,* *Trace Elements and Human Illness*. New York: Praeger, 1980:343–5

152. Tobin DJ, Fenton DA, Kendall MD. Ultra-structural observations on the hair bulb melanocytes in acute alopecia areata. *J Invest Dermatol* 1990;94:803–7

153. Messenger AG, Bleehan SS. Alopecia areata: light and electron microscopic pathology of the regrowing white hair. *Br J Dermatol* 1984; 110:155–62

154. Madani S, Shapario J. Alopecia areata update. *J Acad Dermatol* 2000;42:549–62

Leg, foot and nail disease in the elderly 5

M. Alam, R. K. Scher and P. I. Schneiderman

AGE-RELATED SKIN CHANGES

While facial skin complaints are more frequent, the legs are the second most common site of skin complaints in the elderly[1]. The average duration of these complaints is approximately two years, with the delay in consulting physicians attributed to cost, inconvenience, and a low expectation of improvement[1]. Dermatoses seen on the lower extremities include xerosis, stasis dermatitis, contact dermatitis, cutaneous infections, ulcers, stellate pseudoscars, corns and calluses, tinea pedis and nail dystrophies[1-3]. Etiologically, leg and foot pathology is exacerbated by fat pad atrophy and degeneration of collagen, osteoarthritis-associated problems, impaired circulation, and other systemic diseases[4]. Research into the molecular biology of skin aging is now attempting to clarify mechanisms for chronic damage in both skin that has been exposed to the sun and photoprotected skin[5,6], like the skin of the legs of men. Impairment of the dermal microvasculature and the resulting decreased surface area for nutrient exchange may explain in part poor wound healing in patients with chronic venous insufficiency[7-9]. No general relationship appears to exist between skin thickness and age, but thickness appears to decrease with age in the skin of the extremities[10,11]. Hormone replacement in postmenopausal women may retard this dermal atrophy[12].

STASIS DERMATITIS

Stasis dermatitis has been reported to occur in 6.9% of the elderly[1]. Clinically, stasis dermatitis presents as a red, edematous, eczematous, wet eruption on the bilateral lower extremities that may be acute or chronic, with associated lichenification, hyperpigmentation, fibrotic and atrophic skin and scars over healed ulcers (Figure 1)[3]. Stasis may be differentiated from fungal infection by potassium hydroxide (KOH)-treated scrapings and fungal culture. Recurrent episodes of worsened stasis may be stimulated by self-excoriation and associated infection[13].

Treatment

Treatment for stasis dermatitis requires addressing the underlying peripheral vascular disease and venous stasis, which cause tissue hypoxia, as well as treating the dermatoses[13]. The best treatment plans rely on a team of health-care workers, including the primary physician, vascular surgeon, dermatologist and dermatology nurse-educator. To improve venous outflow, prolonged standing should be avoided and legs should be elevated six or more inches above the heart when the patient is not walking[14]. 'Contour' style reclining chairs (e.g. La-Z-Boy Inc.) may be helpful. A vascular surgery evaluation should be requested to quantify arterial and venous insufficiency and assess the need for surgical treatment of varicosities or other vascular structures. Cardiopulmonary and renal function should be optimized, and hypoalbuminemia corrected[14].

Compression of the legs provides clinical improvement, but should not be attempted until after vascular surgery has checked the patient for arterial insufficiency with Doppler ankle-brachial indices (ABIs) or other indicated testing[15]. All self-administered compression devices should be placed upon arising in the morning and before dependency leads to more swelling. Graduated compression stockings deliver 20–60 mmHg pressure at the ankles and decrease this gradually to nominal compression at the top of the stocking. For normally shaped legs, the ready-to-wear stockings may provide an adequate fit at less expense than custom-made stockings. Packets for patient education can be obtained from the manufacturers. Wearing silk or nylon understockings can allow stockings to slip on more easily and rubber gloves may aid in application by providing a better grip. Zippered stockings are available for those who prefer their ease of use, and stocking removal may be facilitated by using a shoehorn under the cuff of the stocking. Knee high support stockings are preferable to higher stockings since they do not impede popliteal blood flow during flexure. Branching or rolling of stockings should be minimized to avoid a torniquet effect. Since stockings typically last only 3–6 months, frequent replacement is necessary. Patients may prefer to own two pairs at a time so that one may be worn while the other is being laundered[13,14].

Other compression devices can be employed. Elastic bandages (e.g. ACE, Jobst) take longer to apply than stockings and are bulkier, but they are also less expensive. Elastic bandages lose effectiveness after 6–8 months and should be used with caution in arterial insufficiency. Patients with latex allergy can benefit from the recent availability of 100% cotton bandages. Anti-embolism stockings (e.g. TED) create lower compressive pressure than graduated compression stockings and are designed to prevent thrombi and emboli in post-surgical, non-ambulatory patients[13,14]. Pneumatic compression stockings are expensive and may be appropriate for severe cases; they can increase the rate of healing five-fold over that achieved with graduated compression stockings alone[16]. Unna boots are discussed in the section on ulcers.

In addition to compression, topical treatment may be of benefit[13,14]. Patients should be instructed on refraining from rubbing and scratching. Cool compresses, or cool saline or 2.5% Burow's solution soaks, may relieve oozing and blistering. Lubricants, especially bland emollients like petrolatum, should be used at least twice a day to moisten the skin. Anti-inflammatory treatment with topical steroids should be used with caution since application to ulcers may impede healing. In general, medium-strength fluorinated steroids (e.g. triamcinolone 0.1%) can be used twice a day unless severe exacerbation necessitates stronger preparations. Topical antipruritic agents and topical antibiotic preparations should be used sparingly to minimize the risk of allergic contact dermatitis. Auto-eczematization, or 'id' reaction, can occur as a pruritic dermatitis on the face, neck and body as a result of severe stasis dermatitis of the lower extremities[13]. Id reaction may occur in one-third of patients with stasis[17] and will persist until the stasis is controlled, possibly with a 1–2 week course of 40 mg/day of prednisone or by hospitalization for intensive treatment.

CONTACT DERMATITIS

Patch-testing in elderly patients with stasis dermatitis reveals a 60% incidence of at least one positive patch result[18]. Topical treatments applied to areas of chronic ulceration are the most common cause of allergic contact dermatitis of the legs[19,20]. Id reaction may occur at distal body sites. The risk of allergic contact dermatitis may be reduced by limiting the use of topical preparations of questionable efficacy[19]. Significantly, stasis dermatitis in the elderly presents atypically, with relatively less vesiculation and inflammation, more scaling, and earlier onset of severe pruritus, hyperpigmentation and lichenification. Contact dermatitis in the elderly is more persistent and resistant to treatment[3].

Once contact dermatitis is diagnosed, the offending substance should be removed and moderate- to high-potency topical steroids applied twice a day. Oral antihistamines, as well as compresses, may be beneficial, and some authors prefer oral systemic corticosteroid treatment rather than topical corticosteroids to prevent further skin irritation[3,21].

Agents implicated in stasis-associated allergic contact dermatitis include neomycin, epoxy resin[18], lanolin[19], aloe vera[22,23], topical fusidic acid[24] and parabens.

ULCERS

Lower extremity ulcers are common in the elderly and derive from age-related skin changes, peripheral vascular disease and concomitant medical problems (Figures 2–4)[25]. Since 1980 there has been an increased prevalence of pressure ulcers in patients discharged from hospitals[26,27]. Almost two-thirds of pressure ulcers observed in nursing home patients are now present at the time of admission to these facilities[26].

Venous ulcers, which account for 60–70% of all leg ulcers[28], are seen in middle-aged and elderly women. Venous ulceration results from superficial venous insufficiency and may be worsened by thrombosis triggered by external injury[29,30]. Clinically, a bluish-red color precedes the formation of an ulcer usually no more than 3–4 cm in diameter located on the lower medial calf. Superinfection with *Staphylococcus aureus* is frequent[31,32], with resistant staphylococci and *Pseudomonas aeruginosa* infecting the wounds of many hospitalized patients[33]. In proximity to the ulcers, edema, induration, eczematous change and lipodermatosclerosis may be evident[29]. Venous ulcers have a chronic, relapsing course. Ill-advised attempts at self-treatment, and patient apathy and neglect may protract healing time[29]. Patient education should be combined with investigation and treatment of organic causes. Nutritional deficits, including anemia and zinc deficiency[34–42], are seen with regularity in the elderly living alone and require correction. Hemodynamic evaluation should include palpation of pedal pulses, checking of Doppler indices, and elicitation of any history of trauma to the vessels. Work-up for rheumatic or cardiovascular disease may be appropriate, and lesions suspicious for malignancy should be biopsied[29]. Subcutaneous calcification, present in about 10% of patients with chronic venous insufficiency, may be visualized on radiographic film and delay healing[43]. Patients with venous ulcers are easily sensitized to topical allergens[44], and potent topical steroids may inhibit healing. Healing venous ulcers are shallow, have a base of granulation tissue, and display islands of re-epithelialization[29].

Ischemic ulceration due to arterial occlusion also occurs disproportionately in the elderly[45,46]. Arterial ulcers have sharply defined 'punched out' borders and are frequently pretibial or on the toes. They may be more painful that venous ulcers and may not be surrounded by hyperpigmentation or lipodermatosclerosis. Diabetes mellitus, lupus erythematosus, rheumatoid arteritis, poorly applied pressure bandages, burns from hot water bottles and unrelieved pressure on the heels of comatose or paralyzed patients may be predisposing factors for ulcer formation. An improved arterial blood supply secondary to medical or surgical treatment may speed the resolution of ulcers. Excision and skin grafting may be of therapeutic benefit.

Hypertensive ulcers[47–49], more often noted in women, are superficial ulcerations that occur in the presence of peripheral pulses. Livedo may be observed at the site of the ulcers, which have a reddish-yellow edge and are exquisitely painful. Most hypertensive ulcers arise on the anterior aspect of the lower two-thirds of the leg. Trauma may be a causative factor.

Treatment

The treatment of leg ulcers is similar to the treatment of stasis dermatitis in the absence of ulceration. Venous ulcers may also be treated by the application of Unna boots in the physician's office[13,14]. Unna boots are glycerine and zinc oxide bandages that stay in place on the patient's legs for several days. While patients must keep these dressings dry and follow up with regular visits to their physician, the ulcers healing under the dressings are protected from the patient's environment and self-manipulation. Arterial and hypertensive ulcers may be so painful that

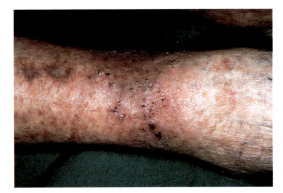

Figure 1 Stasis dermatitis of the lower legs

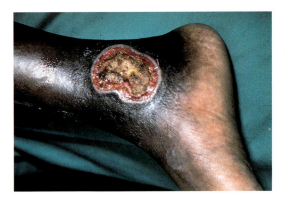

Figure 2 Venous ulcer of the leg

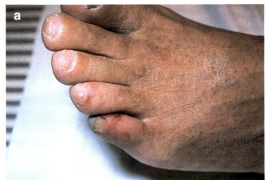

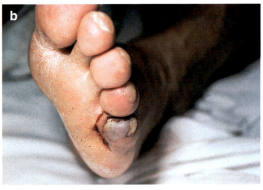

Figure 3 Gangrenous toe secondary to popliteal artery thrombosis

patients require medication for analgesia. Other treatments for lower extremity ulcers include hyperbaric oxygen, skin grafts, and, with accompanying great caution, surgical debridement[29,50–53].

PRURITUS AND XEROSIS

In the elderly, pruritus[2] and xerosis[13] comprise a large portion of all skin complaints. Pruritus, the most common presenting symptom of skin disease in the elderly, can be generalized or localized. Xerosis, like pruritus, can affect the legs focally. Dry, scaly 'winter's itch,' also referred to as asteatotic eczema, involves the lower extremities preferentially. Patients may be urged to wear adequate protective clothing in windy, cold weather. Indoors, they should maintain lower temperatures with the simultaneous use of humidifiers. Decreasing the frequency of bathing and increasing the use of emolliating soaps and moisturizer may relieve both asteatotic eczema and pruritus. Bath oils should be applied with a wet washcloth after the bath to prevent the unsteady patient from slipping in the bathtub or shower. Lactic acid preparations or topical steroids may relieve discomfort in severely scaly and fissured skin of the legs.

FOOT DERMATOSES

An increased emphasis on physical fitness has resulted in an increasing incidence of foot complaints in older patients[4]. Runners, bikers, swimmers and aerobics enthusiasts commonly have foot problems, with 75% of people older than 65 having at least one foot problem requiring medical attention. The regularly seen skin problems include hyperkeratosis,

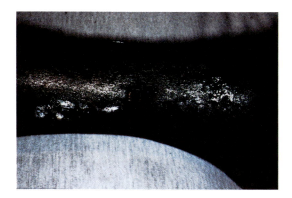

Figure 4 Hypertensive ulcers of the leg

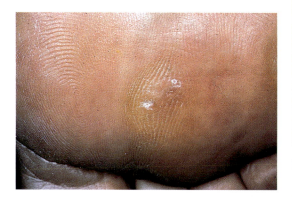

Figure 5 Corns on the foot

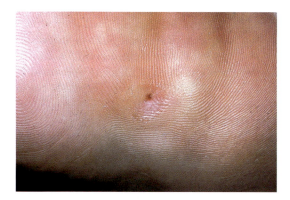

Figure 6 Corn after trimming

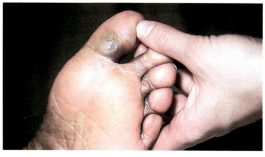

Figure 7 Hemorrhagic callus on the foot

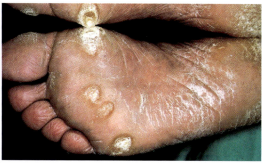

Figure 8 Hereditary painful callosities of the foot

corns and calluses, digital deformities, maceration, infections and nail dystrophies.

Hyperkeratotic lesions (Figures 5–8) occur focally and diffusely over bony prominences and areas of increased friction[54]. Hyperkeratosis is a normal reaction of the skin to internally or externally applied pressure[55] and can present as a callosity, callus, or corn[56]. According to one definition, a callosity is a plaque caused by repeated friction or pressure; a corn is a sharply demarcated callosity over a bony prominence, especially of the hands or feet, that is painful; and a callus is a broad, diffuse hyperkeratosis under the metatarsal heads (Figures 5–8)[57]. Soft corns between the fourth and fifth toes may be extremely painful and accompanied by maceration and cellulitis[58,59]. The soles of the feet in the elderly are vulnerable owing to fat pad atrophy, asymmetric pressure load and impaired vascular supply[60,61]. Hyperkeratoses on the sole can erode to form ulcers, with up to 30% of leg ulcers in the elderly occurring on the foot or sole. In patients with vascular or neurologic impairment, hyperkeratoses should be debrided to see if they conceal a deep ulcer or osseous involvement[54]. For women especially, hyperkeratotic and other foot problems are frequently related to a lifetime of wearing shoes that are too small and narrow[4,62].

Treatment

The treatment[56,63] of hyperkeratotic foot lesions includes assessment and correction of the patient's gait, regular paring, improved shoes, toe separators made of felt, foam, or rubber and other cushioning devices. Petrolatum or 10–20% salicyclic acid preparations may be applied, but irritation should be avoided. As in all foot problems, the failure of pain to remit with conservative treatment should prompt a referral to orthopedic surgery[64,65].

DIGITAL DEFORMITIES

Digital deformities of the feet are hallux valgus (bunion), hallux limitus and hammer toe contractures or claw toes[4,66]. Bunions entail a lateral deviation of the great toe with medial prominence of the metatarsal head at the first metatarsophalangeal joint. Hallux limitus is an osteoarthritis of the first metatarsophalangeal joint. Severe hallux limitus culminates in hallux rigidus, in which the patient finds it difficult to propel the foot forward when walking because of diminished joint motion. Treatments for bunions and related disorders are ice compresses, wider shoes, shoes stretched by a shoemaker, bunion shields and surgery. With hallux limitus, conservative treatment may be of limited benefit. Like bunions, hammer toe contractures and claw toes are exacerbated by narrow shoes. Hammer toe contractures result from the hyperflexion of small toes and the resulting curling of the toes. With age, increasingly rigid and painful contractures occur in association with hyperkeratotic lesions. For relief, patients may try moleskin, corn pads, toe splints, lamb's wool, open toe shoes and emolliation. Severe claw toes and hammer toes may require surgical correction.

Responsible care of the foot in the elderly is based on early and careful attention to problems. If hyperkeratotic lesions become erosive, debridement coupled with padding and polo rings may be appropriate[60,61]. Nurse-educators and physical therapists should be consulted early in the course of foot treatment to help the patient understand self-administered techniques that may enhance symptom reduction. Shoe selection is particularly important yet often overlooked[4,54]. Shoes should have firm soles, soft uppers, good shock absorption properties and proper fit. Sneakers or running shoes are normally sufficient, provided they are replaced often, and custom shoes may be needed only in exceptional circumstances. Absorbent socks protect the foot from shoes and reduce maceration. Acrylic socks may be superior to cotton socks in mitigating blister formation. Closed-cell neoprene insoles are available over-the-counter and may be useful for augmenting the plantar fat pads. As previously noted, dermatologic problems of the foot may be associated with deeper pathology that is best managed by early referral to podiatry or orthopedic surgery. In elderly patients with multiple medical problems, prescription of non-steroidal anti-inflammatory drugs and other medications for pain relief should be discussed with the patient's internist.

INFECTIONS

When foot hyperkeratosis and maceration persist, infection may ensue. Foot infections[66] usually originate in the nail plate or interdigital web spaces. Lower extremity infections are one of the most common reasons for hospital admission of diabetic patients. Typically, these diabetics are in their fifth decade, have had Type II diabetes for about twenty years, and stay in hospital for a month. The natural history of diabetics undergoing above-the-knee or below-the-knee amputations is dismal, with two-thirds dying within five years of surgery[67]. Treatment of diabetic foot infections is foot elevation, rest, local tissue debridement as necessary, and broad-spectrum antibiotics[68–70]. A two-week or longer antibiotic course is standard, and the choice of agent and route of administration should be guided by the patient's local environment, the nature of the initial injury, and the specific microorganisms within the wound; in the hospital, an infectious diseases consultation should be

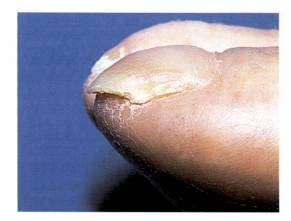

Figure 9 Nail plate with increased longitudinal and transverse curvature

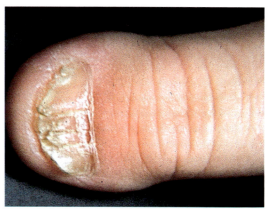

Figure 12 Severely brittle nail with splitting and cracking. Coexisting distal interphalangeal joint osteoarthritis

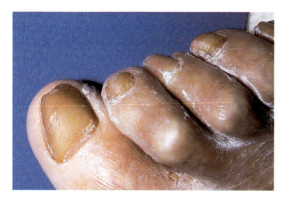

Figure 10 Thickened, yellow nail plate secondary to faulty biomechanics from bony abnormalities of the toes

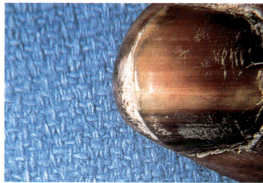

Figure 13 Distal subungual onychomycosis of the hallux with *in situ* melanoma secondary to melanonychia striata

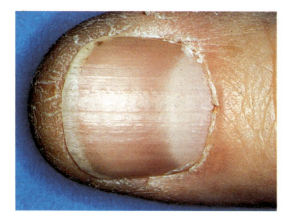

Figure 11 'Beading' of the nail plate with xerotic eczema of periungual skin

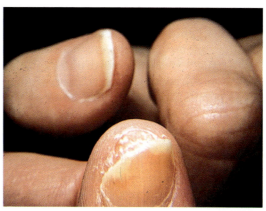

Figure 14 Bowen's disease of the nail bed presenting with distal onycholysis

obtained to clarify medication strategy. The cleaning of the wound should be done with normal saline and isotonic soaps, and dressings and antibiotic ointment can speed granulation. For outpatients, a total contact walking cast, changed weekly, may help by redistributing weight, immobilizing the limb, protecting the wound, reducing edema, and limiting patient involvement in wound care[66].

Other foot and leg infections may be less severe. Toe web maceration may be suspicious for erythrasma[54], a superficial *Corynebacterium minutissimum* infection that displays pink-red fluorescence when illuminated by a Wood's light. Onychomycosis may be accompanied by secondary bacterial infection[54]. Palpating the areas between adjacent metatarsal heads may reveal pain and erythema suggestive of such secondary infection. For small uncomplicated wounds, bland ointments like bacitracin may be cost-effective. Topical neomycin should be avoided to reduce the risk of sensitization, and topical mupirocin should be substituted for use in polymicrobial wounds or shallow wounds in immunocompromised patients[71].

Antibiotic-resistant organisms are becoming an increasing problem in both community-acquired and hospital-related infections, and these may be difficult to eradicate even with multiple systemic agents. Methicillin-resistant *Staphylococcus aureus* (MRSA) infections[72], for instance, are a significant source of morbidity and mortality in elderly patients. Apart from advancing age, risk factors include the presence of open wounds and decubitus ulcers.

Scabies epidemics occur regularly in nursing homes and chronic care hospitals[73–77]. In the elderly and bedridden, scabies infestations present atypically[78], with clumps of red papules sometimes seen more on the trunk than on the extremities. Misdiagnoses include psoriasis, eczema and contact dermatitis. Important predisposing factors are senile dementia, lack of cutaneous sensation, immunosuppression and poor hygiene. Usually the patient who is the vector for spreading scabies in a care facility has a case of keratotic (Norwegian) scabies. In addition to the standard whole body treatment with scabicides, patients should have their nail plates cut short and scabicide applied to their digital tips.

AGE-RELATED NAIL CHANGES

The nails change in appearance over time[79–83]. In the elderly, the nail may be lusterless and opaque, from yellow to gray in color, and with a diminished or missing lunula. The transverse convexity of the nail is more marked, and the longitudinal curvature decreased. Flattening of the nail plate (platonychia), and spooning (koilonychia), are often seen, and these may be accompanied by clubbing of the digit[84–87]. Characteristic color and texture patterns are associated with underlying anemia, renal or hepatic disease and other systemic illnesses[88].

Aging causes a reduction in the linear growth rate of the nail[89–92]. The rate declines steadily from the second decade, and by the end of life is decreased by about 40%. Significantly, the treatment duration for onychomycosis may be correspondingly lengthened in the elderly since treatment efficacy is related to the replacement of infected nail plate by newly produced nail. In addition to growing more slowly, the nail in the elderly is more prone to splitting, fissuring and developing superficial longitudinal furrows, or onychorrhexis[93–95]. Cosmetic improvement of onychorrhexis may be achieved by buffing the nail regularly with a gently abrasive powder, paste, or cream formulation[96,97]. Fingernails tend to soften with age, and toenails to become thicker and more rigid[98]. Pachyonychia, generalized thickening of the nail, may be improved by buffing, or, in severe cases, by chemically or mechanically mediated nail avulsion[99–108]. Intractable cases may require nail matrix destruction. Before an elderly individual is subjected to even a minor surgical procedure, a thorough preoperative assessment of surgical risk should be obtained[109].

Older patients, especially women, may be troubled by age-related increasing brittleness of the nail plate[110,111]. Brittleness may manifest as longitudinal and horizontal ridging, roughness (trachyonychia) and breaks and unevenness at the distal edge of the nail. Treatment entails minimizing repeated cycles of wetting and drying the nail as well as limiting the use of nail enamels and removers[112]. Lactic acid formulations, such as a 12% preparation under occlusion, may be useful moisturizers. Oral biotin may also be of benefit in some cases[113,114]. If nail lacquers are applied to protect the nail, these should not contain formaldehyde[115] and should be used at most once a week.

NAIL UNIT INFECTIONS

Fungal, bacterial and viral infections of the nail unit are prevalent in the elderly. Onychomycosis[116,117], which is relatively more common in the elderly, can be diagnosed by a KOH preparation, a fungal culture of the nail bed and plate, or, most definitively, by a periodic acid-Schiff (PAS)-stained biopsy specimen of the nail[118,119]. The four types of onychomycosis[120-122] are distal subungual, the most common variety, which manifests as subungual hyperkeratosis and lifting of the nail plate; proximal subungual, the least common type, in which a white patch extends from the proximal nail fold to the proximal nail plate; white superficial, which appears as a powdery white accumulation on the surface of the nail; and *Candida* onychomycosis, which is frequently associated with onycholysis and a yellow discoloration of the nail plate. Widely used topical antifungals, including the allylamines and imidazoles, treat tinea pedis but do not clear onychomycosis. If topicals alone are prescribed, they should be applied twice a day for at least 6–12 months, with monthly evaluation and routine nail care[81]. Oral fluconazole, terbinafine, and itraconazole have now been shown to be effective in treating onychomycosis[123-135]. These systemic agents have various dosing regimens, and drug interactions and the risk of hepatic inflammation should be considered and discussed with the patient before they are given. Confirming onychomycosis by KOH, culture, nail clipping histology, or biopsy is recommended before initiating oral treatment. If only one or two nails are markedly dystrophic, nail avulsion[136-138] may be combined with a briefer duration of medical therapy[139].

Bacterial infection of the nail unit may be acute or chronic[81,140]. Acute bacterial paronychia may be prurulent, induced by staphylococcus infection, and treated by incision and drainage followed by oral antibiotics. Chronic paronychia appears as red, edematous, tender nail folds, and may be caused by Gram-negative organisms like *Proteus* or *Klebsiella* species, or by *Candida*. Chronic paronychias may deform the nail plate. The nails should be kept dry and treated with a topical antifungal lotion in addition to a topical antiseptic at least twice a day[141]. Several weeks to months of treatment may be required. The green discoloration of the nail plate caused by *Pseudomonas aeruginosa* infection can be corrected by removing the onycholytic nail plate and applying topical gentamicin or sulfacetamide three times a day[141,142].

Viral infections of the distal digits may not be any more common in the elderly than in other adults[81,143-148]. However, the relative immunosuppression of an elderly patient may suggest the need for more aggressive treatments for such problems as periungual verrucae and herpetic whitlow.

NAIL DYSTROPHIES

Nail unit dystrophies (Figures 9–12) are extremely common and troublesome in the elderly[81]. These include onychauxis, onychoclavus, onychocryptosis, onychogryphosis and onychophosis. Onychauxis refers to localized hypertrophy of the nail plate. Repeated partial debridement of the nail plate or thinning with drills or burs may suffice to produce an adequate cosmetic result. As with severe pachyonychia, severe onychauxis may require chemical or surgical nail avulsion. Onychoclavus denotes a subungual corn under the distal edge of the great toenail. The nail can be clipped back and the lesion removed, with subsequent use of cushioning

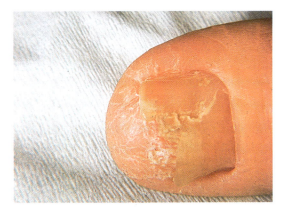

Figure 15 Squamous cell carcinoma of the nail bed with onycholysis and subungual debris

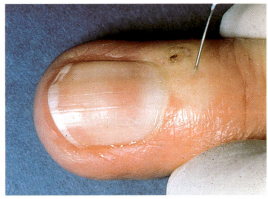

Figure 18 Intralesional corticosteroid treatment of a myxoid cyst

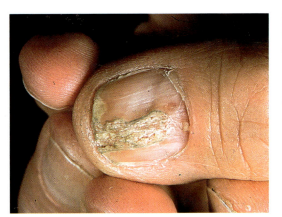

Figure 16 Verrucous squamous cell carcinoma of the nail bed that resembles a wart

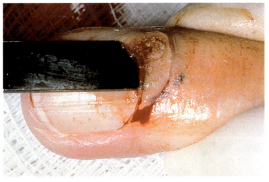

Figure 19 Excision of the proximal nail fold for recalcitrant myxoid cyst

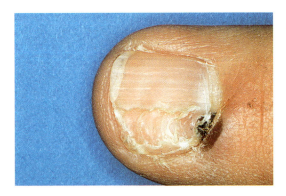

Figure 17 Myxoid cyst of the proximal nail fold with a long groove of the nail plate (focal mucinosis)

pads and comfortable shoes. Underlying osseous deformities may require correction in some instances. Onychocryptosis[149,150], or ingrown nails, may result from poor nail cutting technique or shoes that do not fit[151,152]. If allowed to remain uncorrected, onychocryptosis can result in invasive infection, necrosis, and osteomyelitis. Treatment should consist of cutting the affected nail plate straight across, and placing a piece of cotton under the lateral free edge of the nail to elevate it. Warm soaks may be applied in conjunction with topical or systemic antibiotics. Some practitioners advocate liquid nitrogen cryotherapeutic treatment of the inflamed tissue and ingrown margins[153]. A specially designed wire nail brace can be applied to the ingrown toenail; subsequent tightening of this brace at regular intervals may straighten the nail[154]. Severe cases should be screened by radiographs to rule out osteomyelitis and may need partial or total nail avulsion or matrix ablation. Onychogryphosis, also called ram's horn deformity of the great toenails, arises from self-neglect or the debilitated, elderly patient's inability to care for the nails. Infrequent trimming leads to the formation of large and eccentric nail plates. In acute cases, the affected nail may be filed manually or mechanically into a more regular shape; avulsion or matricectomy may be necessary if conservative treatment fails. Plans should be made for the provision of adequate nail care in the future to forestall a recurrence. Finally, onychophosis entails the development of focal or diffuse hyperkeratotic plaques around the nail unit. Debridement with keratolytics, including 12% lactic acid, 20% urea, and 6–20% salicyclic acid preparations, is indicated. Aggressive emolliation may be prophylactic.

Nail dystrophies may be associated with a patient's other medical problems. As mentioned before, renal and hepatic disease can cause characteristic nail changes. Onychodystrophy has also been observed in a range of diseases that, while not unique to the elderly, are more common in older individuals. For instance, nail dystrophy has been reported in patients with carpal tunnel syndrome[155], multiple myeloma[156], and end-stage renal disease requiring peritoneal dialysis[157]. Unilateral nail changes have been noted after spinal cord injuries[158]. Treatment of the nails in these cases should address functional and cosmetic deficiencies, if any.

Splinter hemorrhages, trauma-related black lesions under the distal two-thirds of the nail, are common in the elderly[81,159]. Like subungual hematomas, splinter hemorrhages arise easily in patients who are anticoagulated, unsteady on their feet, or prone to injury. The incidence of both these lesions can be reduced by avoiding trauma. Acute subungual hematomas[81,160], which are red and tender in contrast to the blue-black, asymptomatic older lesions, may require a simple surgical release. A needle may be used to pierce the overlying nail to relieve the pressure underneath.

CUTANEOUS MALIGNANCIES

While the elderly are often afflicted with persistent stasis dermatitis, ulcerations and foot dermatoses, unremitting dermatologic complaints may indicate the presence of a malignancy (Figures 13–16). Appropriate vigilance is necessary to evaluate such lesions in a timely manner. Any chronic ulceration, irrespective of etiology, may potentially undergo malignant degeneration[54]. Venous stasis ulcers are the most likely to transform into tumors, particularly squamous cell carcinomas (SCCs), and malignant change within a pre-existing ulcer is associated with a poor prognosis[32,54,161]. Primary malignancies of the leg presenting as an ulcer are thought to be more common than malignant degeneration of a previously benign lesion, and primary cancers are also less aggressive. Basal cell carcinomas (BCCs) erupting on the legs may be flat and thus initially undetected[28]. Carcinoma cuniculatum, a rare low-grade type of SCC that displays aggressive local behavior, usually occurs on the soles but has been described in several cases as affecting the toe-nails[162]. Primary SCC of the nail fold may mimic a paronychium[163]. There is considerable evidence confirming the occurrence of BCCs and SCCs in patches and plaques of long-standing stasis[164]. Of course, benign neoplasms, such as myxoid cysts of the digits, are more commonly seen (Figures 17–19).

While ulcers, injuries and stasis are known to be associated with BCCs and SCCs, the data regarding malignant melanoma are sparse. There are a few isolated reports of malignant melanoma developing within stasis dermatitis. Such melanomas may be difficult to identify clinically and histologically, and immunostaining with S-100 protein is imperative. If lesions that appear to be chronic subungual hematomas persist for a lengthy interval, they should be biopsied to rule out melanoma[81]. Other less common tumors have been described on the lower extremities of older patients. Leukemia cutis in chronic myelogenous leukemia has been found to masquerade as stasis dermatitis[165], and subungual metastases from visceral tumors such as breast cancer have been known to resemble acute paronychia of a single toenail[166].

In general, a low threshold for biopsy may be appropriate in elderly persons, particularly those who are fair-skinned. Paronychias, subungual hematomas, venous ulcers and suspicious leg nodules and papules that are persistent should be sampled. Unfortunately, in the context of stasis-related vascular compromise, biopsy sites may be slow to heal. The pervasive scarring, hyperkeratosis and hyperpigmentation seen on the legs of the elderly may also make difficult the delineation of a suspicious lesion embedded within. Dermatologists should use appropriate clinical judgment to weigh the benefits of biopsy against the risk of creating a non-healing wound at a poorly vascularized anatomic location.

PREVENTIVE CARE

Regular skin care can curtail the extent of lower extremity skin disease in the elderly. As much as one half of older patients rely on someone else, usually either a podiatrist or a family member, for routine foot care[1]. Although some may be unable to participate in their own health maintenance, patient education has been shown to be of value in encouraging preventive behaviors. It has been estimated that 50% of amputations in diabetic patients could be avoided by screening and appropriate education[167]. Diabetic patients, as well as those with severe stasis, vascular compromise and ulceration, should be taught to do foot exams according to a prescribed schedule[168]. Primary care physicians and nurse-educators can perform a vital function by administering simple non-invasive screening tests to further assess risk and alert the medical team to the need for intervention[169]. Such screening exams should include palpation and observation of the entire foot and web spaces. Plantar and dorsal surfaces should be checked for protective sensation with a 10-g monofilament, and current footwear should be inspected for proper fit and shape. If practical, ABIs should be obtained with a hand-held Doppler. Nurses may find contact with patients' feet distasteful and may consequently avoid it[170]. Their co-operation may be elicited by reviewing the large body of evidence that confirms the value of routine foot screening and patient education in reducing lower extremity complications[171–173].

FUNCTIONAL AND PSYCHOLOGICAL CONSIDERATIONS

In some instances psychiatric and neurologic disabilities might disqualify the elderly patient from self-care activities. Dementia staging may be obtained by administering the global deterioration scale (GDS), the functional assessment staging measure (FAST), and similar tests[174]. Analysis of gait and verification of the adequacy of extrinsic factors, such as the lighting in the home, may yield information that can be used to lessen the likelihood of falls and lacerations[175]. Patients who are apathetic about their lower extremity pathology, like non-healing ulcers, may benefit from psychiatric consultation[29].

While lower extremity dermatologic problems in the elderly may be acute medical issues or primarily cosmetic concerns, the latter category is not trivial. Outward appearance is important since interpersonal behavior is reciprocal[176]. Indeed, in one study when panelists were shown photographs of people who had aged well or poorly, the attractive group was perceived as exhibiting many positive attributes unrelated to physical appearance[177]. Self-esteem and social confidence in the elderly may thus be enhanced by caregivers' prompt attention to complaints about the appearance of their legs, feet, or nails. Onychomycosis has already been shown to affect quality of life[178]. While patients should be reassured, optimism regarding cosmetic enhancement should be tempered with an acknowledgement of the irreversibility of certain age-related skin changes[179].

References

1. Beauregard S, Gilchrest BA. A survey of skin problems and skin care regimens in the elderly. *Arch Dermatol* 1987;123:1638–43
2. Thaipisuttikul Y. Pruritic skin diseases in the elderly. *J Dermatol* 1998;25:153–7
3. Beacham BE. Common dermatoses in the elderly. *Am Fam Physician* 1993;47:1445–50
4. Gordon GM, Cuttic MM. Exercise and the aging foot. *South Med J* 1994;87:S36–S41
5. West MD. The cellular and molecular biology of skin aging. *Arch Dermatol* 1994;130:87–95
6. Whitmore SE, Levine MA. Risk factors for reduced skin thickness and bone density: possible clues regarding pathophysiology, prevention, and treatment. *J Am Acad Dermatol* 1998; 38:248–55
7. Pappas PJ, DeFouw DO, Venezio LM, *et al.* Morphometric assessment of the dermal microcirculation in patients with chronic venous insufficiency. *J Vasc Surg* 1997;26:784–95
8. Kelly RI, Pearse R, Bull RH. The effects of aging on the cutaneous microvasculature. *J Am Acad Dermatol* 1995;33:749–56
9. Gerstein AD, Phillips TJ, Rogers GS, *et al.* Wound healing and aging. *Dermatol Clin* 1993; 11:749–57
10. Fenske NA, Lober CW. Structural and functional changes of normal aging skin. *J Am Acad Dermatol* 1986;15:571–85
11. Gniadecka M, Jemec GBE. Quantitative evaluation of chronological ageing and photoaging *in vivo*: studies on skin echogenicity and thickness. *Br J Dermatol* 1998;139:815–21
12. Callens A, Vaillant L, Lecomte P, *et al.* Does hormonal skin aging exist? A study of the influence of different hormone therapy regimens on the skin of postmenopausal women using non-invasive measurement techniques. *Dermatology* 1996;193:289–94
13. Walther RR, Harber LC. Expected skin complaints of the geriatric patient. *Geriatrics* 1984; 39:67–80
14. Torrence BP, Hovanec R, Bartunek C. Stasis dermatitis: practical pearls for the dermatologic nurse. *Dermatol Nurs* 1993;5:186–91
15. Zimmet SE. Treatment of stasis dermatitis and ulceration. *Am Fam Physician* 1994;49: 1080, 1083
16. Pekanmaki K, Kolari PJ, Kiistala V. Intermittent pneumatic compression treatment for post-thrombotic leg ulcers. *Clin Exp Dermatol* 1987;12:350–3
17. Stoltze R. Dermatitis medicamentosa in eczema of the leg. *Acta Derm Venereol* (Stockh) 1966;46:54–64
18. Shupp DL, Winkelmann RK. The role of patch testing in stasis dermatitis. *Cutis* 1988;42: 528–30
19. Hogan DJ. Widespread dermatitis after topical treatment of chronic leg ulcers and stasis dermatitis. *CMAJ* 1988;138:336–8
20. Fisher AA. *Contact Dermatitis*. Philadelphia: Lea & Febiger, 1986:92
21. Falanga V. Venous ulceration. *J Dermatol Surg Oncol* 1993;19:764–71
22. Shoji A. Contact dermatitis in *Aloe arborescens*. *Contact Dermatitis* 1982;8:164–7
23. Nakamura T, Kotajima S. Contact dermatitis from *Aloe aborescens*. *Contact Dermatitis* 1984; 11:51
24. Ritchie IC. Antibiotic treatment of soft tissue infections. *Lancet* 1973;1:544
25. Pieper B, Templin TN, Dobal M, *et al.* Wound prevalence, types, and treatment in home care. *Adv Wound Care* 1999;12:117–26
26. Taler G. Management of pressure ulcers in long-term care. *Adv Wound Care* 1997;10:50–2
27. Smith DM, Winsemius DK, Besdine RW. Pressure sores in the elderly: can this outcome be improved? *J Gen Intern Med* 1991;6:81–93
28. Lagattolla NRF, Burnard KG. Chronic venous disease may delay the diagnosis of malignant ulceration of the leg. *Phlebology* 1994;9:167
29. Ryan TJ, Burnand K. Diseases of the veins and arteries: leg ulcers. In Champion RH, Burton JL, Burns DA, Breathnach SM, eds. *Rook/Wilkinson/Ebling Textbook of Dermatology*, 6th edn. Oxford: Blackwell Science, 1998: 2228–75
30. Hjelmstedt A. Bergvall U. Incidence of thrombosis in patients with tibial fractures. *Acta Chir Scand* 1968;134:209–18
31. Phillips TJ, Dover JS. Leg ulcers. *J Am Acad Dermatol* 1991;25:965–87
32. Pennel TC, Hightower F. Malignant changes in post-phlebitic ulcers. *South Med J* 1965;58: 779–81
33. Mitchell AAB, Pettigrew JB, MacGillvray D. Varicose ulcers as reservoirs of hospital strains of *Staph. Aureus and Pseudomonas pyocyanea. Br J Clin Pract* 1970;24:223–6
34. Greaves M, Boyde TRC. Plasma-zinc concentrations in patients with psoriasis, other dermatoses and venous leg ulceration. *Lancet* 1967;ii:1019–20
35. Greaves MW, Ive FA. Double-blind trial of zinc sulphate in the treatment of chronic venous leg ulceration. *Br J Dermatol* 1972;87:632–4
36. Greaves MW, Skillen AW. Effects of long-continued ingestion of zinc sulphate in patients

with venous leg ulceration. *Lancet* 1970;ii: 889–91

37. Myers MB, Cherry G. Zinc and healing of chronic leg ulcers. *Am J Surg* 1970;120:77–81

38. Sergeant GR, Galloway RE, Gueri MC. Oral zinc sulphate in sickle-cell ulcers. *Lancet* 1970; ii:891–2

39. Pories WJ, Henzel JH, Rob CG, *et al.* Acceleration of wound healing in man with zinc sulphate given by mouth. *Lancet* 1967; i:121–4

40. Hallbook T, Lanner E. Serum-zinc and healing of venous ulcers. *Lancet* 1972;ii:780–2

41. Husain SL. Oral zinc zulphate in leg ulcers. *Lancet* 1969;i:1069–71

42. Andrews M, Gallagher-Allred C. The role of zinc in wound healing. *Adv Wound Care* 1999; 12:137–8

43. Lippman HI, Goldin RR. Subcutaneous ossification of the legs in chronic venous insufficiency. *Radiology* 1960;74:279–88

44. Malten KE, Kuiper JP. Allergie cutanée de contact dans 100 cas d'ulcères variqueux. *Phlebologie* 1974;27:417–20

45. Browse NL. Diseases of the heart and blood vessels. Ischaemia of the lower limbs. *Br Med J* 1996;2:157

46. Eastcott HHG. Chronic ischaemia. *Proc R Soc Med* 1962;55:596–9

47. Martorell F. Hypertensive ulcer of the leg. *Angiology* 1950;1:133–40

48. Alberti JMZ. Hypertensive ulcers: Martorell's ulcer. *Phlebology* 1988;3:139

49. Pasyk KA, Thomas SV, Hassett CA, *et al.* Regional differences in capillary density of the normal human dermis. *Plast Reconstr Surg* 1989;83:939–45

50. Tibbs D. *Varicose Veins and Related Disorders*, 2nd edn. Oxford: Butterworth-Heinemann, 1997

51. Thomas S. *Wound Management and Dressings*. London: The Pharmaceutical Press, 1990: 1–211

52. Browse NL, Burnand KG, Lea TM, *et al.*, eds. *Diseases of the Veins: Pathology, Diagnosis and Treatment*. London: Edward Arnold, 1988

53. Compression hosiery for stasis disorders. *Drug Therapy* 1988;297:1159

54. Kosinski M, Ramcharitar S. In-office management of common geriatric foot problems. *Geriatrics* 1994;49:43–9

55. Helfand AE. Nail and hyperkeratotic problems in the elderly foot. *Am Fam Physician* 1989; 39:101–10

56. Kennedy CTC. Mechanical and thermal injury: callosities, corns, and calluses. In Champion RH, Burton JL, Burns DA, Breathnach SM, eds. *Rook/Wilkinson/Ebling Textbook of Dermatology*, 6th edn. Oxford: Blackwell Science, 1998:891–3

57. Singh D, Bentley G, Trevino SG. Callosities, corns and calluses. *Br Med J* 1996;312: 1403–6

58. Gibbs RC, Boxer MC. Abnormal biomechanics of feet and their cause of hyperkeratoses. *J Am Acad Dermatol* 1982;6:1061–9

59. Sarafian SK, ed. *Anatomy of Foot and Ankle*. Philadelphia: Lippincott, 1983:375

60. Bureau Y, Barriere H. Ulcerating and mutilating trophic lesions of the lower limbs. *Br J Dermatol* 1958;70:372–7

61. Andersson E, Hansson C, Swanbeck G. Leg and foot ulcers. An epidemiologic survey. *Acta Derm Venereol* (Stockh) 1984;64:227–32

62. Giannestras NJ. *Foot Disorders: Medical and Surgical Management*. Philadelphia: Lea and Febiger, 1976

63. Abboud RJ, Rowley DI. Foot pressure measurement: history and development. In Helal B, Rowley DI, Crachiolo IIIA, Myerson M, eds. *Surgery and Disorders of the Foot and Ankle*. London: Martin Dunitz, 1996:123–38

64. Regnauld B, ed. *The Foot*. Berlin: Springer-Verlag, 1986

65. Helal B, Rowley DI, Crachiolo IIIA, Myerson MS, eds. *Surgery and Disorders of the Foot and Ankle*. London: Martin Dunitz, 1996

66. Bridges RM Jr, Deitch EA. Diabetic foot infections: pathophysiology and treatment. *Surg Clin North Am* 1994;74:537–55

67. Penn I. The impact of diabetes mellitus on extremity ischemia. In Kempczinski RF, ed. *The Ischemic Leg*. Chicago: Year Book Medical Publishers, 1985:56–9

68. Arcieri G, Griffith E, Gruenwaldt G, *et al.* Ciprofloxacin: an update on clinical experience. *Am J Med* 1987;82:381–6

69. Ingram C, Eron LJ, Goldenberg RJ, *et al.* Antibiotic therapy of osteomyelitis in out patients. *Med Clin North Am* 1988;72:723–38

70. Lipsky BA, Pecoraro RE, Larson SA, *et al.* Outpatient management of uncomplicated lower-extremity infections in diabetic patients. *Arch Intern Med* 1990;150:790–7

71. Ward RS, Saffle JR. Topical agents in burn and wound care. *Phys Ther* 1995;75:526–38

72. Bradley SF. Methicillin-resistant *Staphylococcus aureus* in nursing homes: epidemiology, prevention, management. *Drugs Aging* 1997; 10:185–98

73. Estes SA, Estes J. Therapy of scabies: nursing homes, hospitals, and the homeless. *Semin Dermatol* 1993;12:26–33

74. Witkowski JA. Scabies: subungual areas harbor mites. *J Am Med Assoc* 1984;252:1318–9

75. Scher RK. Subungual scabies. *Am J Dermatopathol* 1983;5:187–9

76. Scher RK. Subungual scabies [Letter]. *J Am Acad Dermatol* 1985;12:577–8

77. DePaoli RT, Marks VJ. Crusted (Norwegian) scabies: treatment of nail involvement [Letter]. *J Am Acad Dermatol* 1987;17:136–9

78. Yonkosky D, Ladia L, Gackenheimer L, *et al.* Scabies in nursing homes: an eradication program with permethrin 5% cream. *J Am Acad Dermatol* 1990;23:1133–6

79. Cohen PR, Scher RK. Geriatric nail disorders: diagnosis and treatment. *J Am Acad Dermatol* 1992;26:521–31

80. Cohen PR, Scher RK. Nail changes in the elderly. *J Geriatr Dermatol* 1993;1:45

81. Cohen PR, Scher RK. The nail in older individuals. In Scher RK, Daniel CR III, eds. *Nails: Therapy, Diagnosis, Surgery*, 2nd edn. Philadelphia: WB Saunders, 1997:127–50

82. Baran R, Dawber RPR. The ageing nail. In Fry L, ed. *Skin Problems in the Elderly*. Edinburgh: Churchill Livingstone, 1985:315–30

83. Cohen PR. The lunula. *J Am Acad Dermatol* 1996;34:943–56

84. Stone OJ, Maberry JD. Spoon nails and clubbing: review and possible structural mechanisms. *Tex Med* 1965;61:620–7

85. Stone OJ. Spoon nails and clubbing: significance and mechanisms. *Cutis* 1975;16: 235–41

86. Stone OJ. Clubbing and koilonychia. *Dermatol Clin* 1985;3:485–90

87. Crosby DL, Petersen MJ. Familial koilonychia. *Cutis* 1989;44:209–10

88. Horan MA, Puxty JA, Fox RA. The white nails of old age (neapolitan nails). *J Am Geriatr Soc* 1982;30:734–7

89. Williams DD, Short R, Bowden DM. Fingernail growth rate as a biomarker in the pigtailed macaque (*Macaca nemestrina*). *Exp Gerontol* 1990;25:423–31

90. Bean WB. Nail growth: thirty-five years of observation. *Arch Intern Med* 1980;140:73–6

91. Hamilton JB, Terada H, Mestler GE. Studies of growth throughout the lifespan in Japanese: growth and size of nails and their relationship to age, sex, heredity, and other factors. *J Gerontol* 1955;10:401–15

92. Balin AK, Pratt LA. Physiological consequences of human skin aging. *Cutis* 1989; 43:431–6

93. Silver H, Chiego B. Nails and nail changes: II. Modern concepts of anatomy and biochemistry of the nails. *J Invest Dermatol* 1940; 3:133–42

94. Ronchese F. Peculiar nail anomalies. *Arch Dermatol* 1951;63:565–80

95. Baran R, Dawber RPR. The nail in childhood and old age. In Barab R, Dawber RPR, eds. *Diseases of the Nails and their Management*, 2nd edn. Oxford: Blackwell Scientific, 1994: 81–96

96. Scher RK. Cosmetics and ancillary preparations for the care of nails: composition, chemistry, and adverse reactions. *J Am Acad Dermatol* 1982;6:523–8

97. Engasser PG. Nail cosmetics. In Scher RK, Daniel CR III, eds. *Nails: Therapy, Diagnosis, Surgery*, 2nd edn. Philadelphia: WB Saunders, 1997:276–81

98. Edelstein JE. Foot care for the aging. *Phys Ther* 1988;68:1882–6

99. Farber EM, South DA. Urea ointment in the non-surgical avulsion of nail dystrophies. *Cutis* 1978;22:689–92

100. South DA, Farber EM. Urea ointment in the nonsurgical avulsion of nail dystrophies – a reappraisal. *Cutis* 1980;25:609–12

101. Buselmeier TJ. Combination urea and salicyclic acid ointment nail avulsion in nondystrophic nails: a follow-up observation. *Cutis* 1980;25:397, 405

102. Dorn M, Kienitz T, Ryckmanns F. Onychomycosis: experience with nontraumatic nail avulsion. *Hautarzt* 1980;31:30–4

103. Hardjoko FS, Widyanto S, Singgih I, *et al.* Treatment of onychomycosis with a bifonazole-urea combination. *Mycoses* 1990;33: 167–71

104. Hay RJ, Roberts DT, Doherty VR, *et al.* The topical treatment of onychomycosis using a new combination urea/imidazole preparation. *Clin Exp Dermatol* 1988;13:164–7

105. Torres-Rodriguez JM, Madrenys N, Nicolas MC. Non-traumatic topical treatment of onychomycosis with ureas associated with bifonazole. *Mycoses* 1991;34:499–504

106. Sears JK. The use of a combination nail elevator and hemostat clamp: new instruments for nail avulsion. *J Dermatol Surg Oncol* 1992; 18:223–5

107. Ceilley RI, Collison DW. Matricectomy. *J Dermatol Surg Oncol* 1992;18:728–34

108. Miller MA, Brodell RT. The treatment of the splitting nail with phenol alcohol partial nail matricectomy. *Dermatol Surg* 1996;22:388–90

109. Duncan KO, Leffell DJ. Preoperative assessment of the elderly patient. *Dermatol Clin* 1997;15:583–93

110. Scher RK. Brittle nails. *Int J Dermatol* 1989; 28:515–16

111. Lubach D, Cohrs W, Wurzinger R. Incidence of brittle nails. *Dermatologica* 1986;172:144–7

112. Wallis MS, Bowen WR, Guin JD. Pathogenesis of onychoschizia (lamellar dystrophy). *J Am Acad Dermatol* 1991;24:44–8

113. Colombo VE, Gerber F, Bronhofer M, Floersheim GL. Treatment of brittle fingernails and onychoschizia with biotin: scanning electron microscopy. *J Am Acad Dermatol* 1990;23:1127–32

114. Hochman LG, Scher RK, Meyerson MS. Brittle nails: patient response to daily biotin supplementation. *Cutis* 1993;51:303–5

115. Kechijian P. Geriatric nail disorders [Letter]. *J Am Acad Dermatol* 1993;28:133–4

116. Scher RK. Onychomycosis: a significant medical disorder. *J Am Acad Dermatol* 1996;35:S2–5

117. Machler BC, Kirsner RS, Elgart GW. Routine histologic examination for the diagnosis of onychomycosis: an evaluation of sensitivity and specificity. *Cutis* 1998;61:217–9

118. Cohen PR, Scher RK. Nail disease and dermatology [Commentary]. *J Am Acad Dermatol* 1989;21:1020–2

119. Haneke E. Fungal infections of the nail. *Semin Dermatol* 1991;10:41–53

120. Baran R, Hay RJ, Tosti A, *et al*. A new classification of onychomycosis. *Br J Dermatol* 1998;139:567–71

121. Zaias N. Onychomycosis. *Arch Dermatol* 1972;105:263–72

122. Norton LA. Nail disorders: a review. *J Am Acad Dermatol* 1980;2:451–67

123. Bootman JL. Cost-effectiveness of two new treatments for onychomycosis: an analysis or two comparative clinical trials. *J Am Acad Dermatol* 1998;38:S69–72

124. Elewski BE. Onychomycosis: pathogenesis, diagnosis, and management. *Clin Microbiol Rev* 1998;11:415–29

125. Elewski BE, Hay RJ. Update on the management of onychomycosis: highlights of the third annual international summit on cutaneous antifungal therapy. *Clin Infect Dis* 1996;23:305–13

126. Epstein E. How often does oral treatment of toenail onychomycosis produce a disease-free nail. An analysis of published data. *Arch Dermatol* 1998;134:1551–4

127. Gupta AK, De Doncker P, Scher RK, *et al*. Itraconazole for the treatment of onychomycosis. *Int J Dermatol* 1998;37:303–8

128. Gupta AK, Scher RK. Fluconazole for the treatment of onychomycosis: an update. *Int J Dermatol* 1998;37:815–20

129. Katz, HI. Systemic antifungal agents used to treat onychomycosis. *J Am Acad Dermatol* 1998;38:S48–52

130. Leyden J. Pharmacokinetics and pharmacology of terbinafine and itraconazole. *J Am Acad Dermatol* 1998;38:S42–7

131. Shuster S. Onychomycosis: making sense of the assessment of anti-fungal drugs. *Acta Derm Venereol* (Stockh) 1998;78:1–4

132. Tosti A, Piraccini BM, Stinchi C. Relapses of onychomycosis after successful treatment with systemic antifungals: a three-year follow-up. *Dermatology* 1998;197:162–6

133. Zaias N. Management of onychomycosis with oral terbinafine. *J Am Acad Dermatol* 1990;23:810–2

134. Meinhof W. Kinetics and spectrum of activity of oral antifungals: the therapeutic implications. *J Am Acad Dermatol* 1993;29:S37–41

135. Roseeuw D, DeDoncker P. New approaches to the treatment of onychomycosis. *J Am Acad Dermatol* 1993;29:S45–50

136. Rollman O, Johansson S. *Hendersonula toruloidea* infection: successful response of onychomycosis to nail avulsion and topical ciclopiroxolamine. *Acta Derm Venereol* (Stockh) 1987;67:506–10

137. Hettinger DF, Valinsky MS. Treatment of onychomycosis with nail avulsion and topical ketoconazole. *J Am Podiatr Med Assoc* 1991;81:28–32

138. Geronemus RG. Laser surgery of the nail unit. *J Dermatol Surg Oncol* 1992;18:735–43

139. Korting HC, Schafer-Korting M. Is tinea unguium still widely incurable? A review three decades after the introduction of griseofulvin. *Arch Dermatol* 1992;128:243–8

140. Elewski BE. Bacterial infection in a patient with onychomycosis. *J Am Acad Dermatol* 1997;37:493–4

141. Wilson JW. Paronychia and onycholysis, etiology and therapy. *Arch Dermatol* 1965;92:726–30

142. Gunnoe RE. Diseases of the nails: how to recognize and treat them. *Postgrad Med* 1983;74:357–62

143. Lim JTE, Goh CL. Carbon dioxide laser treatment of periungual and subungual viral warts. *Australas J Dermatol* 1992;33:87–91

144. Kuflik EG. Specific indications for cryosurgery of the nail unit. Myxoid cysts and periungual verrucae. *J Dermatol Surg Oncol* 1992;18:702–6

145. Rampen FHJ, Steijlen PM. Diphencyprone in the management of refractory palmoplantar and periungual warts: an open study. *Dermatology* 1996;193:236–8

146. Holland TT, Weber CB, James WD, *et al*. Tender periungual nodules. Myrmecia (deep palmoplantar warts). *Arch Dermatol* 1992;128:105–6, 108–9

147. Gibson JR, Harvey SG. Interferon in the treatment of persistent viral warts. *Dermatologica* 1984;167:47–8

148. Shumer SM, O'Keefe EJ. Bleomycin in the treatment of recalcitrant warts. *J Am Acad Dermatol* 1983;9:91–6

149. Siegle RJ, Stewart R. Recalcitrant ingrowing nails. Surgical approaches. *J Dermatol Surg Oncol* 1992;18:744–52

150. Ikard RW. Onychocryptosis. *J Am Coll Surg* 1998;187:96–102

151. Lloyd-Davies RW, Brill GC. The aetiology and outpatient management of ingrowing toenails. *Br J Surg* 1963;50:592–7

152. Mortimer PS, Dawber RPR. Trauma to the nail unit including occupational sports injuries. *Dermatol Clin* 1985;3:415–20

153. Sonnex TS, Dawber RPR. Treatment of ingrowing toenails with liquid nitrogen spray cryotherapy. *Br Med J* 1985;291:173–5

154. Dawber RPR, Baran R. Nail surgery. In Samman PD, Fenton DA, eds. *The Nails in Disease*. London: William Heinemann, 1986: 194–206

155. Romani J, Puig L, de Miguel G. Carpal tunnel syndrome presenting as sclerodactylia, nail dystrophy and acro-osteolysis in a 60-year-old woman. *Dermatology* 1997;195: 159–61

156. Mancuso G, Fanti PA, Berdondini RM. Nail changes as the only skin abnormality in myeloma-associated systemic amyloidosis [Letter]. *Br J Dermatol* 1997;137:471–2

157. Caputo R, Gelmetti C, Camiaghi S. Severe self-healing nail dystrophy in a patient on peritoneal dialysis. *Dermatology* 1997;195: 274–2

158. Harris AJ, Burge SM, Gardener BP. Unilateral nail dystrophy after C4 complete spinal cord injury [Letter]. *Br J Dermatol* 1996;135:855–7

159. Young J, Mulley G. Splinter haemorrhages in the elderly. *Age Ageing* 1987;16:101–4

160. Seaberg DC, Angelos WJ, Paris PM. Treatment of subungual hematomas with nail trephination. A prospective study. *Am J Emerg Med* 1991;9:209–10

161. Schraibman IG. The bacteriology of leg ulcers. *Phlebology* 1987;2:265

162. Tosti A, Morelli R, Fanti PA, *et al*. Carcinoma cuniculatum of the nail apparatus: report of three cases. *Dermatology* 1993;186:217–21

163. Hochman LG. Paronychia: more than just an abscess. *Int J Dermatol* 1995;34:385–6

164. Blessing K. Malignant melanoma in stasis dermatitis. *Histopathology* 1997;30:135–9

165. Butler DF, Berger TG, Rodman OG. Leukemia cutis mimicking stasis dermatitis. *Cutis* 1985;35:47–8

166. Cohen PR, Buzdar AU. Metastatic breast carcinoma mimicking an acute paronychia of the great toe: case report and review of subungual metastases. *Am J Clin Oncol* 1993;16:86–91

167. Boulton AJM. Why bother educating the multi-disciplinary team and the patient – the example of prevention of lower extremity amputation in diabetes. *Patient Educ Couns* 1995;26:183–8

168. Frykberg RG. Epidemiology of the diabetic foot: ulcerations and amputations. *Adv Wound Care* 1999;12:139–41

169. Rice KL, Chambers PW. Amputation in the diabetic population: not necessarily a given. *Today Surg Nurse* 1997;19:31–6

170. Richbourg MJ. Preventing amputations in patients with end stage renal disease: whatever happened to foot care? *Anna J* 1998; 25:13–20

171. Caputo GM, Cavanaugh PR, Ulbrecht JS, *et al*. Assessment and management of foot disease in patients with diabetes. *New Engl J Med* 1994;321:854–60

172. Maldonato A, Bloise D, Ceci M, *et al*. Lessons from patient education. *Patient Educ Couns* 1995;26:57–66

173. Litzelman DK, Slemenda CW, Langefeld CD, *et al*. Reduction of lower extremity clinical abnormalities in patients with non-insulin dependent diabetes mellitus. *Ann Intern Med* 1993;119:36–41

174. Reisberg B, Sclan SG, Franssen E, *et al*. Dementia staging in chronic care populations. *Alzheimer Dis Assoc Disord* 1994;8: S188–205

175. Teresi J, Lawton P, Ory M, *et al*. Measurement issues in chronic care populations: dementia special care. *Alzheimer Dis Assoc Disord* 1994; 8:S144–83

176. Kligman AM, Koblenzer C. Demographics and psychological implications for the aging population. *Dermatol Clin* 1997;15:549–53

177. Graham J, Kligman AM. Physical attractiveness, cosmetic use and self-perception in the elderly. *Int J Cosmetic Sci* 1985;7:85

178. Drake LA, Scher RK, Smith EB, *et al*. Effect of onychomycosis on quality of life. *J Am Acad Dermatol* 1998;38:702–4

179. Cook JL, Dzubow LM. Aging of the skin. Implications for cutaneous surgery. *Arch Dermatol* 1997;133:1273–7

Superficial mycoses in the elderly

6

B. P. Glick, M. Zaiac, G. Rebell and N. Zaias

INTRODUCTION

As the world's population continues to age and our patients are exposed to various environmental changes, newer antimicrobial therapies, immunosuppressive drugs and cancer chemotherapeutic agents, physicians will become more likely to face the challenge of treating superficial mycoses.

Superficial mycoses are fungal infections that affect primarily the nonliving, cornified layer of skin, hair and nails. Dermatophytosis, also known as 'ringworm' or tinea and non-dermatophyte infections caused by *Candida albicans* and other yeasts (referred to as dermatomycoses) typically involve truncal, scalp, intertriginous and glabrous skin, and, at times, the external components of the eye including the eyelids, eyelashes, eyebrows, and, rarely, the conjunctivae[1]. Superficial fungal infections responsible for cutaneous diseases in the elderly include dermatophytosis, tinea versicolor and cutaneous candidiasis and its variants. This chapter reviews the clinical, diagnostic and histologic features of superficial fungal disease and discusses appropriate management of these infections in the geriatric population.

DERMATOPHYTOSIS

Definition

The dermatophytes are a group of taxonomically related fungi capable of colonizing keratin-containing tissues such as the stratum corneum of the epidermis, nails, hair, the horny tissues of various animals and the feathers of birds[2]. Keratinophilic fungi may be divided into three categories derived from an ecologic perspective and are known as geophilic (soil derived), zoophilic (animal derived) and anthropophilic (human derived) fungi. The three genera responsible for dermatophyte infections in humans are *Trichophyton*, *Microsporum* and *Epidermophyton*. Of these, *Trichophyton* species are responsible for the overwhelming majority of dermatophyte infections in the elderly. The most common dermatophytic species and the diseases they cause are presented in Table 1.

Although many species of dermatophytes have been identified, only a small number are responsible for the development of disease in humans[3]. Geophilic fungi have adapted for habitation in the soil. Humans are affected sporadically and the most common offending agent is *Microsporum gypseum*.

Zoophilic organisms primarily infect higher animals but may be sporadically transmitted to humans. While zoophilic superficial fungal infections have typically occurred from animal sources in rural areas, infections transmitted from domestic animals and pets have become increasingly common in urban and suburban areas. Transmission may occur by direct animal contact, or indirectly by fomites via infected animal hairs carried on clothes or, in the rural setting, contaminated farm structures such as stalls, barns or animal feed[3].

Anthropophilic species have developed through adaptation away from the soil or animal reservoirs and directly infect humans. Transmission of these organisms occurs human-to-human by direct contact or indirectly by fomites. In contrast to zoophilically derived infections, which suppurate in exposed areas (e.g. face, beard, scalp), anthropophilic organisms tend to produce a non-inflammatory reaction, often located

Table 1   The dermatophytes and their syndromes

Species source	Clinical type	Comments
Microsporum canis (zoophilic/cat)	Fluorescent tinea capitis and isolated lesions on glabrous skin; juveniles and young females	Related epidemic anthropophilic species now rare
Trichophyton tonsurans (Anthropophilic)	Nonfluorescent tinea capitis and isolated lesions on glabrous skin; juveniles and adult females	Chronic in some adult females and related species; *T. violaceum*, *T. soudanense*
Trichophyton mentagrophytes (zoophilic/rodents, rabbits, other mammals)	Tinea capitis and isolated lesions on glabrous skin; all ages	Inflammatory; interdigital tinea pedis is common in the elderly
Trichophyton verrucosum (zoophilic/cattle)	Tinea capitis and isolated lesions on glabrous skin and intertriginous skin; all ages	Inflammatory; including tinea barbae
Trichophyton equinum (zoophilic/horse)	Isolated lesions on glabrous skin; all ages	
Trichophyton rubrum (anthropophilic)	Chronic tinea pedis, manus, cruris, corporis and onychomycosis; all ages	Commonest cause of dermatophytosis; chronic tinea pedis usually presents as a primary infection
Microsporum gypseum (geophilic/garden soil)	Tinea capitis and isolated lesions on glabrous skin; all ages	

on covered areas such as the feet and groin. Differences in susceptible host responses or strain virulence, however, make marked inflammatory reactions (e.g. kerion formation) possible in anthropophilic species[3].

In our geriatric population host defenses play an important role in the epidemiology of anthropophilic infections. Patients with underlying disease states that impart immune suppression are likely to demonstrate dermatophytosis that is more severe and recalcitrant to treatment. In general, factors such as age, sex, race, habits, geographic location, travel history and genetic background[4] may also represent host differences and ultimately affect the progression of disease and the response to treatment.

Clinical features

The earliest lesion of dermatophytosis presents as a small vesicle that is surrounded by inflammation. As this primary lesion grows peripherally, the vesicle ruptures, ultimately leaving a collarette of scale and the typical annular, tinea or 'ring-like' lesion of dermatophyte infection (Figure 1). In some cases only one arc or part of the ring is visible (Figure 2).

As a result tinea corporis is often misdiagnosed as some other dermatologic condition, such as allergic contact or nummular dermatitis, and the patient is treated with topical corticosteroids. The undisclosed dermatophyte infection ultimately produces a 'butterfly-like' lesion or biconcentric rings, representing a steroid-exacerbated dermatophyte infection, and unmasks the so-called 'tinea incognito' (Figure 3). Direct microscopic examination of scales from the affected areas reveals multiple branched and septate hyphae (fungal elements) typical of these superficial fungal infections (Figure 4).

Diagnosis

The presumptive diagnosis of superficial fungal or dermatophyte infections should be supported by direct microscopy of clinical material and confirmed by culture of a specimen on a suitable mycologic medium[5]. The technique of direct microscopic examination depends largely on the dermatologic location of the superficial fungus and should only include keratinaceous (stratum corneum) material. Specimens for direct microscopic examination are taken from the active borders of a lesion or from collarettes of scale by scraping with the dulled edge of a scalpel or clean glass slide and are deposited onto the microscope slide. A cover slip is then placed over the keratinaceous debris and a drop of a clearing solution such as 20% potassium hydroxide (KOH) with dimethylsulfoxide (DMSO) is placed at the edge of the cover slip/slide interface. The solution should flow evenly under the cover slip by surface tension. Clearing solutions such as KOH with DMSO are used to obviate the need for heat fixing and enhance the digestion of epidermal proteins, lipids and debris[5]. A positive, direct microscopic KOH preparation is characterized by branching and septate hyphal elements. This indicates only the presence of fungus. Confirmation of the specific offending agent may be achieved by culture using a suitable medium.

Culture and culture media

Culture identification of the dermatophytic etiology depends specifically on the microscopic, macroscopic and, in some circumstances, the physiologic characteristics of the organism. To identify the etiologic agent, an appropriate, preferably selective culture medium is necessary for adequate growth of the organism (Figure 5). Non-selective media such as Sabouraud's agar do not select for the growth of fungi, and saprophytic overgrowth is common[6,7].

Management

Treatment of dermatophyte infections includes control of local and environmental factors such as moisture and temperature as well as the use of topical and systemic antimycotic therapies. Single or few lesions of tinea infection can best be treated by topical antifungal creams or gels, which tend to serve as a drying agent. Currently available topical antimycotic therapies include topical azoles (e.g. ketoconazole, econazole, oxiconazole and others), ciclopirox olamine, allylamines, (e.g. naftifine, terbinafine) and the newer benzylamines

(e.g. Mentax®). Azoles are fungistatic and are applied b.i.d. typically for 2 to 4 weeks. Allylamine and benzylamine antimycotics are fungicidal and provide the advantage of reduced dosing frequency and overall duration of therapy, usually 1 to 2 weeks[8,9].

Widespread lesions, especially those involving the immunocompromised host, often require systemic antifungal therapy. Various medications and their dosing schedules are as follows:

(1) Griseofulvin 500–1000 mg daily in divided doses of the Gris-PEG (ultramicrosize) formulation;

(2) Ketoconazole 200 mg orally daily for 2 weeks (with appropriate monitoring of liver function); and

(3) Newer systemic antimycotic agents, two triazoles (itraconazole and fluconazole) and the allylamines (terbinafine), which are highly effective in the treatment of dermatophytosis. These new generation oral agents have all but replaced griseofulvin and ketoconazole in the current treatment of superficial dermatophyte fungal infections.

Table 2 provides a summary of the definition, diagnosis and treatment of dermatophytosis[10–12].

TINEA VERSICOLOR

Definition

Tinea versicolor, while uncommon in the elderly, is a chronically recurring superficial mycosis of the stratum corneum caused by *Malassezia furfur* and *Pityrosporum* species, lipophilic yeasts considered to be part of the endemic skin flora (Table 3). Currently it appears that *Pityrosporum* species (*P. orbiculare, P. ovale*) are the favored terminology and accepted etiologic agents for tinea versicolor and its variants. The disease is characterized by scaly, hypo- and hyperpigmented, variably shaped macules typically perifollicular in location and may be found on the trunk,

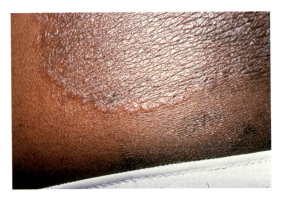

Figure 1 The typical appearance of dermatophyte (tinea) infection is a 'ring-like' or annular lesion as seen in this case of tinea corporis by *T. rubrum*. (Courtesy of M. Zaiac, MD, Mt Sinai Medical Center)

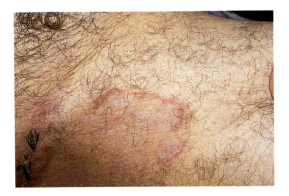

Figure 2 In some cases of dermatophytosis only one arc or portion of the 'ring' is visible. Often the tinea corporis is misdiagnosed as some other cutaneous eruption such as nummular eczema or allergic contact dermatitis. (Courtesy of M. Zaiac, MD, Mt Sinai Medical Center)

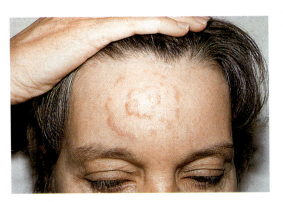

Figure 3 Biconcentric or multiple 'rings' are also a marker for dermatophyte infection exacerbated by the use of topical corticoids. (Courtesy of M. Zaiac, MD, Mt Sinai Medical Center)

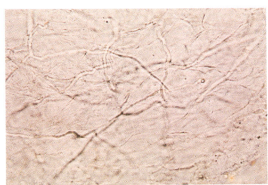

Figure 4 Direct microscopy of keratinaceous debris with 20% KOH with DMSO demonstrating branched and septate hyphae, the hallmark of dermatophyte infections. (Courtesy of B.P. Glick, DO, MPH)

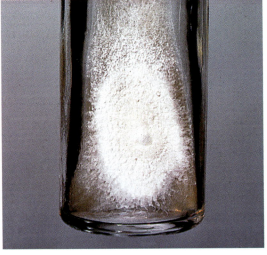

Figure 5 A positive fungal culture demonstrating the presence of dermatophytes caused by *Trichophyton mentagrophytes*. (Courtesy of B.P. Glick, DO, MPH)

neck, face, scalp or proximal extremities (Figure 6)[3]. Tinea versicolor occurs with high prevalence in tropical climates where there are high humidity, high temperatures and frequent exposure to sunlight. All of the clinical variants have an equal sex distribution. While adolescents and young adults are the groups most commonly affected, the elderly are usually affected in special circumstances such as a prolonged occlusion or when in a state of immune suppression[13].

Table 2   Dermatophytosis – key clinical points

Definition
Acute and chronic superficial mycotic infections
caused by the genera *Trichophyton, Microsporum*
and *Epidermophyton*

Dermatologic findings
Reddish scaly papules
Annular lesions
Individual or multiple lesions
May be vesicular
Pruritic

Diagnostic tests
Microscopic examination with potassium
hydroxide (KOH)
Culture in selective medium (e.g. DTM, Mycosel)

Therapy
   Topical antifungal agents
     Azoles
     Triazoles
     Ciclopirox olamine
     Allylamines
     Benzylamines
   Systemic agents
     Ketoconazole 200 mg q.d.
     Fluconazole 100–200 mg q.d.
     Itraconazole 200 mg b.i.d.
     Terbinafine 250 mg q.d.
     Griseofulvin 250–500 mg b.i.d.

Contraindications
Use of corticosteroids

Complications
Secondary bacterial infection
Fungemia (rare)

Prognosis
Good with complete therapy, except in
immunocompromised host

Table 3   Tinea versicolor – key clinical points

Definition
Recurrent superficial infection by *Malassezia furfur*
(*Pityrosporum* sp.)

Dermatologic findings
Pink scaly papules
Greasy plaques
Hypo- or hyperpigmentation
Perifollicular occurrence

Diagnostic tests
Direct microscopic examination of scale (e.g. KOH,
Albert's solution – 'spaghetti and meatballs'
appearance)

Therapy
Ketoconazole 2% shampoo
Selenium sulfide 2.5% shampoo 20 minutes every 2 weeks
Terbinafine 1% spray b.i.d. x 2–4 weeks
or Itraconazole 100 mg b.i.d. for 7 days
Ketoconazole 200 mg p.o. q.d. for 5 days or 400 mg as
a single dose
Fluconazole 400 mg as a single dose

Complications
None

Prognosis
Clearing of acute state
Will recur

Clinical features

Three variations of tinea versicolor by
M. furfur (*Pityrosporum orbiculare, P. ovale*) may
occur:

(1) Papulosquamous lesions;

(2) Folliculitis; and

(3) Inverse tinea versicolor.

On the upper trunk and often extending to
the neck and proximal arms are fine, scaly,
guttate or nummular patches, typically on
individuals who perspire freely. The face,
scalp and genital areas are less frequently
involved. The individual lesions are variable
in their color, ranging from whitish-yellow to

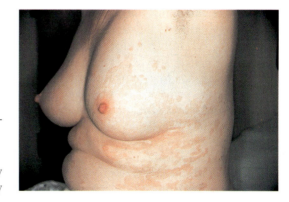

Figure 6   Tinea versicolor may present as hypo- or
hyperpigmented fine, scaly guttate or nummular macules
and patches most commonly located on the upper trunk,
neck and proximal arms. (Courtesy of M. Zaiac, MD,
Mt Sinai Medical Center)

reddish-brown in pale skin, or hypopigmented, fine scaly macules in dark skin. The source
of this hypopigmentation is unclear. However,
ultrastructural studies have demonstrated the
production of abnormally small melanosomes,
decreased numbers of melanosomes and

impaired transfer of these organelles to keratinocytes[14].

The typical presentation of tinea versicolor reflects concern over the appearance of the lesions. Occasionally mild itching and inflammation are present. Other sites of predilection for tinea versicolor include the sternal region, chest, abdomen, back and intertriginous areas. The skin of the palms and soles may also be occasionally involved[15].

Pityrosporum folliculitis is another well recognized clinical entity not infrequently found in the geriatric population. Previously referred to as 'follicular seborrheide'[16], *Pityrosporum* folliculitis is a chronic papulopustular eruption that is more pruritic than tinea versicolor. Sites of predilection for this clinical variant include the chest, upper back and, less frequently, the proximal extremities, face, scalp and sometimes the abdomen. This clinical entity may also be found in association with typical tinea versicolor or seborrheic dermatitis[17]. The primary lesions are 1 to 3 mm follicular and perifollicular erythematous papules and/or pustules. KOH preparation, culture on appropriate medium and, occasionally, a biopsy are required to distinguish this entity from bacterial folliculitides or folliculitis caused by *Candida* species. Predisposing factors to *Pityrosporum* folliculitis include diabetes mellitus and prior corticosteroid and/or antibiotic treatment. Treatment for this clinical sub-type of *Pityrosporum* infection includes selenium sulfide shampoo, 50% propylene glycol in water, topical econazole or ketoconazole cream and, more recently, systemic treatments with ketoconazole, itraconazole or fluconazole[11,12]. Responses vary considerably and the disease often recurs.

Inverse tinea versicolor refers to *Pityrosporum* infection limited primarily to the flexural areas. In these locations the lesions may be confused with seborrheic dermatitis, psoriasis, erythrasma, candidiasis and dermatophyte infection[18].

Diagnosis

Lesions of tinea versicolor that are barely perceptible may be brought readily into view in a darkened room using the Wood's light. The lesions undergo a yellowish or brownish fluorescence that enables the clinician to determine the extent of disease as well as the level of response to therapy. The clinical appearance of tinea versicolor is characteristic, and KOH preparation usually confirmatory. Albert's stain (a combination of malachite green with methylene blue) is also quite helpful in identifying the blunt-edged hyphae and clusters of spores forming the 'spaghetti and meatballs' histological pattern typical of this disease[19].

The technique of obtaining scales from affected areas in *Pityrosporum* infection is identical to that used to diagnose dermatophytosis. Scales may also be removed by using completely transparent Scotch tape and viewing the scales by direct microscopy after application of a clearing solution.

Mycologic culture is rarely performed because of the characteristic appearance of this disease and the ease of diagnosis by KOH preparation. When mycological culture is used, Sabouraud's dextrose agar, overlaid on its surface with olive oil or lanolin, may readily support the growth of this lipohilic yeast-like organism[19].

Etiology

Tinea versicolor occurs owing to infection by *Pityrosporum* species. These organisms are dimorphic, lipophilic and grow *in vitro* in the presence of medium-chain fatty acids. The organisms may convert from yeast to mycelial phases, and it is the mycelial phase that is responsible for clinical disease. Clinical disease with *M. furfur* or *Pityrosporum* sp. occurs under one or some of the following conditions: a warm or humid environment, genetic predisposition, Cushing's disease, diabetes, immunosuppression, and/or malnutrition. Tinea versicolor is therefore an opportunistic infection[20].

Pathology

Because of its clinical presentation and characteristic findings on KOH preparation, biopsy for histologic evaluation of tinea versicolor is rarely necessary. When routine histological sections are evaluated, organisms are usually readily seen in the stratum corneum, and periodic acid–Schiff (PAS) stain is confirmatory. As previously described, although not necessary for diagnosis, *M. furfur* and *Pityrosporum* sp. may be cultured on standard synthetic media, overlaid with a thin layer of sterile olive oil. Within 5 to 7 days at approximately 30°C small, cream-to-tan, yeast-like colonies can be seen. Microscopic evaluation of these colonies reveals budding yeast cells. Hyphae may occasionally be seen[19].

Differential diagnosis

Tinea versicolor must be differentiated from seborrheic dermatitis, pityriasis alba, confluent and reticulate papillomatosis of Gougerot and Carteaud, pityriasis rosea, tuberculoid leprosy, secondary lues and vitiligo. Its characteristic clinical presentations and typical locations in the non-immunocompromised host allow for simple and rapid diagnosis of this condition.

Management

The management of tinea versicolor includes a number of topical and systemic agents that are effective in controlling the disease in the aged. The most common is 2.5% selenium sulfide lotion, which is applied within and around the affected area, left in place for approximately 10–20 minutes and then washed off thoroughly. The process is repeated daily for 2 weeks until clearing, then one to two times per month prophylactically[21]. Numerous dosing schedules for selenium sulfide have been used, each with similar efficacy.

Other topical agents used in the treatment of tinea versicolor include miconazole, tolnaftate, clotrimazole, econazole cream, 25% sodium thiosulfate, salicylic acid soaps and shampoos, keratolytic products, such as 50% propylene glycol and, most recently, terbinafine spray. Systemic agents such as ketoconazole, itraconazole and fluconazole have been used with variable dosing schedules with success[11,12]. Oral terbinafine has not been shown to be effective in adequately clearing this condition. Oral ketoconazole may also be used prophylactically, once or twice per month. When these agents are used with increasing frequency, liver function studies and monitoring should be performed when clinically indicated. Griseofulvin has no activity against *M. furfur* and should not be used.

Course and prognosis

Despite adequate responses to therapy, tinea versicolor is frequently a recurrent disease. Prophylactic measures discussed previously may be helpful in reducing the risk of recurrence.

CANDIDIASIS

Definition

Cutaneous candidiasis and its variants may well be some of the skin diseases most commonly evaluated by geriatricians and dermatologists in the ambulatory, hospital and skilled nursing settings (Table 4).

In general medical terms, the word candidiasis is used to denote infection caused by yeast of the genus *Candida*. From the point of view of the dermatologist, superficial candidiasis of the skin and mucous membranes denotes specific and characteristic syndromes caused by *Candida albicans*, a yeast fungus often found residing as commensal flora in the intestinal tract and frequently as a pathogen in the vaginal tract or in the oral cavity of the immunocompromised host[22].

Clinical features

Ordinary cutaneous candidiasis consists of localized, approximately 1 mm diameter, pustules on erythematous bases, which coalesce to form more widespread erythema and erosions of the stratum corneum and superficial epidermis. Cutaneous candidiasis occurs in moist and intertriginous areas, under conditions of increased temperature and sweating[22]. A classic form is diaper rash in children.

Table 4   Cutaneous candidiasis – key clinical points

Definition
An opportunistic skin and mucous membrane infection
   by *C. albicans*

Dermatologic findings
Individual 1 mm pustules on red skin base
Confluency of pustules/erosions

Diagnostic tests
Gram stain
Germ tube formation and culture

Therapy
Topical polyene (nystatin)
Topical azoles
Topical allylamines
Itraconazole 200–400 mg p.o. q.d.
Fluconazole 150–400 mg p.o. q.d.
Ketoconazole 200–400 mg p.o. q.d.

Complications
Secondary bacterial infection
Rare dissemination

Prognosis
Good with ongoing treatment
Poor in immunocompromised host

In adults, especially the elderly, the toe webs, groin, axillae and inframammary folds are most commonly involved. Inframammary intertrigo is perhaps the most common form of candida infection presenting to the physician and dermatologist (Figure 7). Other areas less commonly involved include the belt line and buttocks. In the toe webs itching, redness and the development of erosions constitute an important episodic or chronic component of the 'athlete's foot' syndrome. In addition, cutaneous candidiasis may be found in occupational skin disease in those patients whose hands are frequently immersed in water or irritated by detergents, resulting in chronic inflammation and infection of the perionychium and interdigital spaces. These findings are especially common in females. As our graying population grows and lives longer, it is probable that more and more geriatric occupational diseases will be seen and it may well be that candida infections become a primary or secondary contributor to occupational skin disorders.

A second form of candidiasis with important dermatologic features is chronic mucocutaneous candidiasis. This occurs in patients with a deficiency of a leukocyte myeloperoxidase and is manifest by severe chronic erosive and crusted lesions of the skin and mucous membranes primarily involving the facial areas[23].

In the immunocompetent host, the facial skin is not usually involved in the common forms of cutaneous candidiasis. Perleche (angular cheilitis), which involves the corners of the mouth and the lips, may be associated with oral candidiasis and does suggest some degree of defect in host resistance (Figure 8)[24]. The most common clinical subtypes of candida infection that affect the elderly include vulvovaginal candidiasis, intertrigo and *Candida* paronychia.

A subtle state of immune suppression, the presence of diabetes or malignancy and undergoing cancer chemotherapy or other immunosuppressive therapies are all settings that can predispose to the development of candida infections in the elderly[22].

Diagnosis

The diagnosis of cutaneous candidiasis consists of direct microscopic examination of cutaneous yeast forms and pseudohyphae as well as isolation of this yeast fungus in culture. For direct examination Gram stain is often preferred, since yeast cells are often difficult to detect in KOH preparations. Wood's lamp fluorescence is usually not helpful, although some data suggest that *Candida* may be adequately detected by autofluorescence[25]. Yeast cells and pseudohyphae are typically Gram-positive. A Giemsa stain or comparable preparation may be very useful for prompt histopathologic diagnosis. For the culture of *C. albicans*, a selective medium containing cyclohexamide as a mycotic and bacterial inhibitor is satisfactory as *C. albicans* is usually resistant. Other yeasts and *Candida* species are, however, to a varying degree, susceptible to cyclohexamide and must be cultured on media without this inhibitor[3].

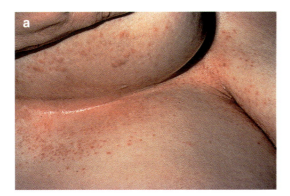

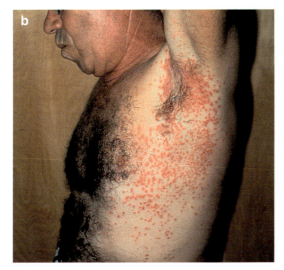

Figure 7 Cutaneous candidiasis. The intertriginous regions of the inframammary folds (a) and axillary creases (b) are two of the most common locations for the development of this superficial mycosis. (Courtesy of the American Academy of Dermatology and M. Zaiac, MD, Mt Sinai Medical Center)

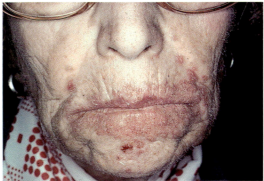

Figure 8 Perleche, a form of angular cheilitis caused by *C. albicans*, involves the corners of the mouth and lips and may be associated with oral candidiasis. (Courtesy of N. Zaias, MD, Mt Sinai Medical Center)

Etiology

The particular significance of *C. albicans* is that it is a normal inhabitant of the intestinal flora, and does not otherwise occur in nature. Candidiasis, therefore, is a commensal organism with the capacity to become an opportunistic pathogen[3]. *Candida albicans* has emerged as the most common and important opportunistic pathogenic fungus. *Candida* does not occur as a natural part of normal human skin flora. However, in the case of typical superficial candidiasis, the organism opportunistically colonizes skin that has become environmentally susceptible to conditions such as increased heat, moisture, occlusion and compression of previously inflamed skin. There is much evidence that a general state of immune deficiency is involved[26]. In addition, an appropriate environment such as an intertriginous fold may accommodate significant amounts of moisture and ultimately provide a setting that leaves the host susceptible to superficial yeast infections. In the case of superficial candidiasis involving the eyelids, conjunctiva and cornea, both local conditions and a generally lowered host resistance may be involved[27]. In the special case of chronic mucocutaneous candidiasis a special defect in leukocyte function has been identified, and in the case of severe host immunodeficiency, *C. albicans* infection may present as a generalized life-threatening mycosis[28]. Hematogenous spread of *Candida* infection resulting in miliary candidiasis may occur. Yeast elements may become lodged in retinal capillaries leading to local endogenous endophthalmitis.

The development of intertriginous and other forms of cutaneous candidiasis in the elderly occurs not only on the basis of local conditions, host resistance and direct infection, but also on the sites of the organisms normally resident in the intestinal tract, vagina and oral cavity. These sites are a common source for infection and reinfection with *C. albicans*.

Treatment

It is apparent from the aforementioned that the treatment of candidiasis is complicated by three factors: (1) the presence of a carrier state of *Candida* in the gastrointestinal tract or vagina; (2) the presence of decreased local resistance of the skin due to heat, moisture and a change in skin integrity; and (3) the presence of a decreased host resistance due to underlying disease.

Cutaneous candidiasis can be treated topically both by means of topical polyenes such as nystatin, or by means of imidazole compounds, that have proven to be highly effective in the treatment of superficial fungal infections[11,12]. Creams and ointments may be used but powders such as nystatin and miconazole (ZeAsorb-AF®) may be used successfully in moist and often macerated intertriginous areas. Other *Candida* infections such as onychomycosis and chronic mucocutaneous candidiasis are notoriously recalcitrant to therapy. Topical and systemic therapy may be required, and the addition of agents such as oral ketoconazole 200–400 mg per day, Sporanox 200–400 mg per day or Diflucan 150–400 mg per day have resulted in dramatic responses to therapy[29–31]. Other oral and intravenous agents used in the treatment of systemic candidiasis include 5-fluorocytosine, amphotericin B, miconazole and clotrimazole[3]. Immunomodulating drugs such as transfer factor, thymosin, cimetidine and levamisole have also been used with limited success[32–34].

Other yeast infections

Other species of the genus *Candida* have been found to occur less frequently in skin disease. Of these, there are several species and variants of medical interest including *C. tropicalis, C. glabrata* (torulopsosis), *C. lusitania,* and *Trichosporon beigelii.* Of these, the only clinically significant dermatologic syndrome is caused by *T. beigelii,* the so-called 'white piedra'. Trichosporosis is an infection of the hair shafts with white nodular elements containing yeast forms, usually found in individuals with poor hygiene[35]. While this condition is rare in the United States, *T. beigelii* is frequently isolated from the skin and nails and may be associated with systemic opportunistic infections involving the skin, internal organs and periocular structures[36].

References

1. Baker RD. *The Pathologic Anatomy of Mycoses.* Dritter band, Funflerteil. Berlin: Springer – Verlag, 1971:211–377
2. Martin AG, Kobayashi GS. Fungal diseases with cutaneous involvement. In Fitzpatrick TB, ed. *Dermatology in General Medicine.* New York: McGraw-Hill, 1999:2337–57
3. Rippon JW. *Medical Mycology: the Pathogenic Fungi and Pathogenic Actinomycetes.* Philadelphia: Harcourt Brace Jovanovich, 1988
4. Blank H, Nann DI, Peale PA. Distribution of dermatophytosis according to age, ethnic group, or sex. *Sabouraudia* 1974;12:352–61
5. Zaias N, Taplin D. Improved preparation for the diagnosis of mycologic diseases. *Arch Dermatol* 1966;93:608–9
6. Rebell G, Taplin D, Blank H. *Dermatophytes: Their Recognition and Identification.* Miami: Dermatology Foundation of Miami, 1964
7. Taplin D, Zaias N, Rebell G, *et al.* Isolation and recognition of dermatophytes on a new medium (DTM). *Arch Dermatol* 1969;99:203–4
8. Bergstresser PR, Elewski B, Zaias N, *et al.* Topical terbinafine and clotrimazole in interdigital tinea pedis: a multicenter comparison of cure and relapse rates with 1 and 4 week treatment regimens. *J Am Acad Dermatol* 1993;28:648–51
9. Lesher JL, Smith JG. Antifungal agents in dermatology. *J Am Acad Dermatol* 1987;17:383–96
10. Stiller MJ, Sangueza OP, Shupack JL. Systemic drugs in the treatment of dermatophytoses. *Int J Dermatol* 1993;32:16–21
11. Gupta AK, Sauder DN, Shear NH. Antifungal agents: an overview. Part 1. *J Am Acad Dermatol* 1994;30:677–98
12. Gupta AK, Sauder DN, Shear NH. Antifungal agents; an overview. Part 2. *J Am Acad Dermatol* 1994;30:911–33

13. Roberts SO. *Pityrosporum orbiculare*: incidence and distribution on clinically normal skin. *Br J Dermatol* 1969;81:264

14. Karauoui R. Tinea versicolor: ultrastructural studies on hypopigmented and hyperpigmented skin. *Dermatologica* 1981;162:69–70

15. Catterall MV. Tinea versicolor: a reappraisal. *Int J Dermatol* 1980;19:84

16. Jillson OF. *Pityrosporum* folliculitis. *Cutis* 1985; 33:226

17. Back O. *Pityrosporum* folliculitis: a common disease of the young and middle-aged. *J Am Acad Dermatol* 1985;12:56

18. Roberts SO. Pityriasis versicolor. A clinical and mycological investigation. *Br J Dermatol* 1969; 81:315

19. Chandler FW, Watts JC, eds. Tinea versicolor. In *Pathologic Diagnosis of Fungus Infections*. Chicago: ASCP Press, 1987:215–17

20. Tanaka M, Imamura S. Immunological studies on *Pityrosporum* genus and *Malassezia furfur*. *J Invest Dermatol* 1979;73:321

21. Albright SD III. Rapid treatment of tinea versicolor with selenium sulfide. *Arch Dermatol* 1966;93:460

22. Smith CB. Candidiasis: pathogenesis, host resistance, and predisposing factors. In Bodey GP, Fainstein V, eds. *Candidiasis*. New York: Raven Press, 1985:53

23. Jorizzo JL. Chronic mucocutaneous candidosis. An update. *Arch Dermatol* 1982;65:431

24. Lehner T. Classification and clinicopathological features of *Candida* infections of the mouth. In Winner HI, Hurey R, eds. *Symposium on Candida Infections*. Baltimore: Williams and Wilkins, 1966:19

25. Margo CE. The diagnostic value of autofluorescence. *Sur Ophthalmol* 1985;29:374–6

26. Synderman R. Defective mononuclear leukocyte chemotaxis: a previously unrecognized immune dysfunction. *Ann Intern Med* 1973; 78:50

27. Montes LP, Wilborn WH. Fungus–host relationship in candidiasis: a brief review. *Arch Dermatol* 1985;121:119

28. Arnold HP, Odom RB, James WD. Systemic candidiasis. In *Andrews' Diseases of the Skin*. Philadelphia: WB Saunders, 1990:345–6

29. Drouhet E, Dupont B. Treatment of chronic mucocutaneous candidiasis and other superficial and systemic mycoses successfully treated with ketoconazole. *Rev Infect Dis* 1980;2:606

30. Burke WA. Use of itraconazole in a patient with chronic mucocutaneous candidiasis. *J Am Acad Dermatol* 1989;21:1309–10

31. Kirkpatrick CH. Chronic mucocutaneous candidiasis. *J Am Dermatol* 1994;31:514

32. Horsmanheimo M, Krohn K, Virolainen M, *et al*. Immunologic features of mucocutaneous candidiasis before and after treatment with transfer factor. *Arch Dermatol* 1979;115:180–4

33. Akhter J, Merker RI, Rieger CH, *et al*. Effect of thymosin on lymphocytes from patients with chronic mucocutaneous candidiasis and endocrinopathies. *J Allergy Clin Immunol* 1980;65: 34–40

34. Jorizzo JL, Sams WM, Jegasothy BV, *et al*. Cimetidine as an immunomodulator: chronic mucocutaneous candidiasis as a model. *Ann Intern Med* 1980;92:192–5

35. Conant NF. *Manual of Clinical Mycology*. Philadelphia: WB Saunders, 1971:632

36. Manzella P, Berman IJ, Kukrika MD. *Trichosporon beigelii* fungemia and cutaneous dissemination. *Arch Dermatol* 1982;118:343–5

Scabies and pediculosis

7

S. P. Stone

INTRODUCTION

The geriatric population is thought to be at particular risk for certain infectious diseases, among them the common infestation with the itch mite, *Sarcoptes scabiei*. Particularly in the institutionalized elderly, scabies not only can cause great anxiety and apprehension among health care workers, but may also be over diagnosed because of the considerable concern for the possibility of epidemics within an institution[1]. Pediculosis, on the other hand, whether the infestation is with scalp lice, body lice or crab (pubic) lice, is not thought to be a particularly significant problem in the elderly.

SCABIES

The epidemiology of this human parasitic infestation is well understood. Scabies (Figure 1, also see Chapter 3, Figure 12) is believed to occur in cycles of approximately ten to thirty years, but appears to have persisted at high levels in the United States and abroad for the past twenty years, with a major increase since 1991[2]. It has become a major problem in nursing homes, particularly in patients who are debilitated and require extensive hands-on nursing care[3]. While very few data exist on the incidence of scabies in home care, it would seem reasonable to assume that there is also a relatively high risk for infestation in such patients.

In dealing with the institutionalized elderly with possible scabies infestation, nursing staff and management are frequently unaware of proper control measures. As a result excessive measures such as quarantine and mass prophylaxis of both patients and the facility staff are often unnecessarily invoked.

Epidemiology and clinical features

Contrary to popular belief scabies is not a disease which recognizes social distinctions; it affects people of all socioeconomic levels, without regard to age, gender, race, or standards of personal hygiene. Transmission of scabies usually requires direct skin-to-skin contact with an infested person. Infrequently, transmission can also occur by contact with clothing or bedding but only if contamination of these articles occurs immediately before contact, for example sharing of bedding or bath towels while still wet. Interestingly, one author, D. Burns, has suggested that multiple cases of scabies in a nursing home or home for the elderly are 'almost invariably associated with the presence of an unrecognized case of crusted (Norwegian) scabies' pointing out that until the index patient is identified and treated, attempts to eradicate the problem may prove unsuccessful[4]. The present author's experience does not support such a blanket statement, but it is clear that one factor facilitating the spread of scabies in the elderly, especially the institutionalized elderly, is a delay in diagnosis. Often this is due to a failure to consider the diagnosis (most probably in non-institutionalized elderly) or to an atypical appearance of the eruption, which indeed may be somewhat different from the classical distribution and morphology.

When the adult female mite, which is only 0.3–0.4 mm (less than 1/50th of an inch) in size, is transferred to the skin of a new host she quickly burrows beneath the epidermis, where she subsequently lays her eggs. These burrows are typically seen as pruritic lesions on the hands, finger webs, wrists, waistline, and anterior and posterior axillary folds; they also are seen on the external genitalia of men, and the nipples, abdomen and lower buttocks of women. After a latent period of two to six weeks during which the patient becomes sensitized to the ova and excreta of the mite, the intense pruritus begins, with the characteristic nocturnal accentuation of itching. Individuals who have previously been infested will develop symptoms only one to four days after re-exposure.

Nodular scabies is a variation wherein the involved site develops into an inflammatory nodule which on biopsy may show mite parts or an inflammatory infiltrate which may simulate Langerhans cell histiocytosis or pseudolymphoma. Pediatric patients may develop lesions of nodular scabies anywhere on the skin, while adults most often develop the nodular lesions on the genitalia.

Crusted or hyperkeratotic scabies, formerly described as Norwegian scabies, is an uncommon variant of this infestation. While in common scabies there are few mites, probably because scratching destroys the burrows, crusted scabies may present with thousands of mites. In crusted scabies, the host's response to the mites is modified, allowing them to multiply. It is most commonly seen in immunosuppressed patients, particularly individuals with acquired immunodeficiency syndrome (AIDS) as well as patients who are immunosuppressed by disease or medical treatment (i.e. with chronic steroids and immunosuppressives (Figure 2)).

Patients with reduced sensation secondary to sensory neuropathy or spinal injury do not perceive itch and therefore do not scratch, but many patients with crusted scabies show no demonstrable sensory loss. In addition to immunosuppressed patients, elderly patients, especially those with dementia, and patients with Down's syndrome as well as other mentally retarded patients are particularly susceptible to crusted scabies. The reason for crusted scabies occurring in patients with mental retardation and neurologic disease (such as stroke patients) is not understood, but some authors have theorized that a reduced itch sensation may be responsible.

Patients with arthritis and other debilitating disease may develop crusted scabies, possibly owing to an inability to scratch themselves. Crusted scabies has also resulted from inappropriate use of potent fluorinated topical steroids[5]. Here, too, the theory is that suppression of itching by the steroid results in less scratching, and thus the mites are not dug out by the fingernails.

Early case recognition and treatment are of primary concern for the prevention of secondary cases and potential epidemic outbreaks. It is not uncommon for health-care workers to acquire occupational scabies, especially on the upper arms and abdomen, but rarely on the hands and wrists.

Diagnosis

The diagnosis is confirmed by the demonstration of mites, eggs or fecal pellets (scybala) on skin scrapings (Figure 3). Burrows should be sought in the areas of common involvement as listed above (hands, finger webs, wrists, waistline and especially the periumbilical area, anterior and posterior axillary folds, external genitalia of men, nipples and lower buttocks of women), and these areas are best examined with a magnifying glass or binocular loupe. The burrows may be 2 to 15 mm in length, straight, curved, S shaped or even L shaped. Because the typical scabies victim probably has fewer than 15 adult mites (various authors say 10, 11 or 12; the point remains valid) on his or her skin at any one time, the mites may be difficult to find, and a negative scraping does not rule out scabies infestation. A drop of mineral oil is placed on the suspicious papule or burrow, and the area is firmly scraped or shaved with a scalpel blade. If there is scaling, as with interdigital involvement, a curette may be used.

Alternative approaches to diagnosis include the epidermal shave biopsy: a superficial shave biopsy using a flexible razor blade, a technique described as simple, essentially painless, and more reliable (Figure 4)[6]. The burrow ink test is also sometimes used to increase test sensitivity. This consists of rubbing a fountain pen or felt tipped marking pen over suspicious areas, wiping the ink off with alcohol, and then examining for burrows highlighted by the remaining ink[7]. A new technique using epiluminescence microscopy with a 40x stereo microscope was recently described as a very useful tool for *in vivo* diagnosis of scabies. The authors described small, dark, triangular structures and a subtle linear segment below the base of the triangle, which was made visible by the presence of small air bubbles. Together, both structures resembled what the authors describe as a 'jet with contrail'. The triangular structure corresponds to the pigmented anterior section of the mite, while the linear segment was thought to be the burrow of the mite along with its eggs and fecal pellets[8].

Pathology

Generally, one would not do a skin biopsy to make the diagnosis of scabies, but occasionally a cutaneous eruption will be biopsied because the diagnosis of scabies was either not entertained or could not be confirmed. Histopathologic findings in the primary scabietic lesion include hyperkeratosis, acanthosis and spongiosis in the epidermis, with some vesiculation. Dermal changes include perivascular and diffuse infiltrates, mainly consisting of mononuclear cells, with a variable number of eosinophils. Increased numbers of mast cells may be seen, slightly more in primary lesions than in secondary lesions and normal skin. Vasculitis has been reported in some cases showing tissue eosinophils, severe dermatitis and many mites. In nodular scabies, there are perivascular infiltrates, primarily histiocytes, some with atypical and hyperchromatic nuclei and a few in mitosis, and some lymphocytes. The secondary lesions may show acanthosis and perivascular inflammatory cell infiltrates, mainly mononuclear cells. Even clinically normal skin showed very slight perivascular and diffuse mononuclear cell infiltrates in half the patients in one study. Circulating levels of eosinophils may be increased, and both the eosinophil count and the serum IgE correlate with the severity of the skin reaction. In one report, 10 out of 60 patients with scabies had markedly increased numbers of circulating eosinophils during scabies infestation, and in most patients levels of circulating eosinophils decreased after scabies treatment[9].

Therapy

The treatment of choice for scabies is 5% permethrin (Acticin®, Bertex Pharmaceuticals, West Virginia; Elimite®, Allergan Inc., California, USA). Unlike earlier treatment modalities such as lindane (Kwell), 5% permethrin has no reported teratogenic or mutagenic effects. A study in *Archives of Dermatology* in 1996 estimated the risk of toxicity as 40 to 400 times greater with lindane than with permethrin[10]. In addition, neurotoxicity has not been reported with 5% permethrin. Permethrin undergoes insignificant absorption, 2% or less in patients with moderate to severe scabies, and is rapidly degraded by esterases to inactive metabolites excreted in the urine[11]. One 60 g tube is generally sufficient for two applications, which should include the entire body from the neck down. Special attention should be paid to the underside of well-trimmed fingernails. The medication should be left on overnight for 8–12 hours and then washed off. According to the package insert, and most clinical studies, one treatment is sufficient. However, because of the possibility of skipping areas of involvement, many dermatologists recommend a second treatment in 5 to 7 days.

In a large multi-center trial which involved 467 patients, a single whole body application of 5% permethrin was compared to an application of 1% lindane. At 4 weeks after treatment (plus or minus 7 days), 91% were cured with permethrin and only 86% with lindane. Interestingly, the pruritus persisted for more than three weeks in 14% of the patients treated with the permethrin product and in 25% of the lindane group[12]. Because of the persistence of itching, the author routinely gives patients 40 to 60 mg of triamcinolone acetonide intramuscularly, or a short course

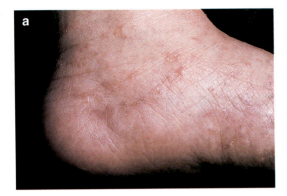

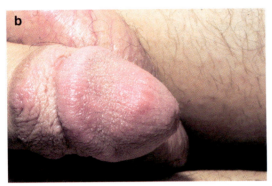

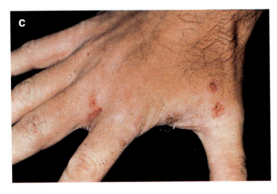

Figure 1   Scabies afflicting the foot (a), the penis (b) and the hand (c)

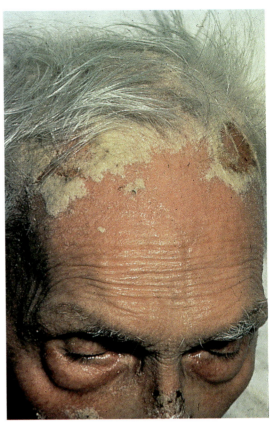

Figure 2   Crusted, or hyperkeratotic, scabies affecting the scalp

of oral steroids, advising them that the steroid would not do anything for their scabies, but would eliminate the itching a week or two sooner than without the steroid.

Other treatments include crotamiton (Eurax) which is less effective as an acaricidal drug, but has the advantage of being anti-pruritic. Multiple treatments are required. Twenty-five per cent benzoyl benzoate is available in Europe but in the United States it must be compounded. Sulfur 3–10% in lotion form and 10% in petrolatum, has been recommended for use in infants, but permethrin is now the treatment of choice even in infants as young as 2 months.

In 1994 ivermectin, an anthelminthic agent in use in much of the underdeveloped world for onchocerciasis and strongyloidiasis, was reported as an effective treatment for scabies[13,14]. Subsequently there have been several reports of the use of ivermectin in the treatment of endemic scabies in nursing homes[15]. Concerns were raised about this modality after an article in the *Lancet* in 1997 reported that in a group of nursing home residents who were treated with ivermectin for an epidemic of scabies on one nursing unit, the number of deaths about six months or more later seemed to be disproportionate to

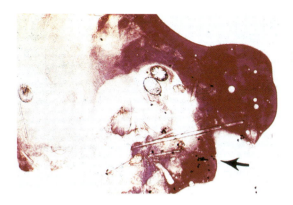

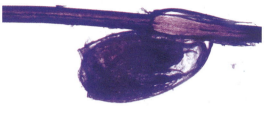

Figure 3 Diagnosis of scabies by low-power view showing several ova and scybala; the arrow points to a collection of these tiny clusters of feces. Figure reproduced with permission from Stone SP. Scabies. *Am Fam Physician* 1977; 15:152–3

Figure 5 Nit (egg of *Pediculus humanus capitis*) cemented to hair shaft

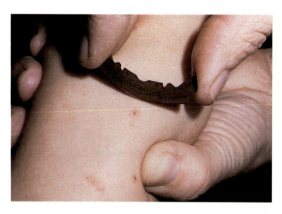

Figure 4 Shaving the papule to remove the intact scabies parasite; a razor blade flexed to the appropriate curvature is the most useful instrument. Figure reproduced with permission from Stone SP. Scabies. *Am Fam Physician* 1977;15:152–3

the deaths in the rest of the nursing home[16]. The correspondence that ensued, as well as subsequent reports, seemed to indicate that the excess deaths were an aberration[17–20].

Ivermectin is a semi-synthetic derivative of *Streptomyces avermitilis*. It is metabolized in the liver and excreted in the feces and in milk. It has a half-life of 12–16 hours and its concentration peaks in the blood at 4 hours. It is neurotoxic to arthropods and nematodes and so is used for a variety of worms. In the United States it is approved for onchocerciasis and strongyloidiasis. It is teratogenic in

mice, rats and rabbits, but only in doses which are toxic to the mother, and so there is some question as to whether this teratogenicity is significant in humans. Side-effects include eosinophilia (3%), hemoglobin increase (about 1%), either pruritus or dizziness (about 3%) and nausea or diarrhea (2%), and a small number of patients have reported anorexia, constipation, vomiting, rash, or tremor in about the same frequency as with doxycycline, tetracycline and aspirin.

The drug is administered in a dose of 200 μg/kg body weight; it is obtained as a scored 6 mg pill so it can be prescribed in multiples of 3 mg. A single dose is effective, although there have been reports in crusted scabies where a second treatment was required a week later, primarily in immunosuppressed and AIDS patients.

Single infestations of scabies in a family are uncommon. Thus, members of the household and sexual contacts should be treated prophylactically. Additional measures for the control of scabies center primarily on early recognition and treatment of cases together with the use of hot water wash and dry cycles for the laundering of contaminated undergarments and bedding which have been in direct contact with the infested patient within the previous 48 hours. Hot water washing, for a minimum of ten minutes, hot air tumble drying, dry cleaning and hot ironing are effective in killing both adult mites and their eggs. Treated health-care workers are considered to be non-infectious after one overnight application of permethrin, and should be allowed to return to work the next day.

Conclusion

The incidence of scabies in the geriatric population will, in general, be far overshadowed by infections with viral, bacterial and fungal organisms. Nonetheless, owing to a prolonged, asymptomatic incubation period and a low index of suspicion on the part of physicians, nursing home and home health workers, scabies can at times cause significant morbidity in both normal and immunocompromised patients. On the other hand, early recognition of potential cases by healthcare personnel and the subsequent implementation of simple and effective control measures can serve to significantly reduce the risk of transmission. In addition, education of all health-care personnel about the true epidemiology of scabies can contribute significantly to lessening undue fear and apprehension associated with what Dr R. Sharbaugh[1] describes as 'this microscopic terrorist'.

PEDICULOSIS

Lice are arthropods belonging to the order Phthiraptera (wingless insects). They include the suborder Anoplura (sucking lice) and the families Pediculidae and Phthiriidae. Two species of lice infest humans, *Pediculus humanus* and *Pthirus pubis* (pubic louse). *Pediculus humanus* is divided into 2 subspecies, *Pediculus humanus capitis* (head louse) and *Pediculus humanus corporis* (body louse). These subspecies have identical morphology, although the body louse tends to be larger, and the subspecies are interfertile. Interestingly, their differences may represent a response to environment: head lice grown on the body acquire the characteristics of body lice and vice versa[21]. Pediculosis refers to infestation with any of these parasites. There are no free-living forms of these insects, and they cannot survive on other animals. Lice are host-specific, and dog lice cannot infest humans, nor will human lice survive on pets.

The life cycles of these lice are fundamentally the same, consisting of adults (male and female), eggs and nymphs. Eggs, or nits, are laid by fertilized females following copulation. The head louse and the pubic (crab) louse glue their eggs to the base of the host's hair, while the body louse attaches its eggs to clothing fibers. The total number of eggs laid per female is variable, reports indicating numbers from 50 to 150 for the human head louse, up to 3000 (Elgart, 1990)[21] for the human body louse, and from 20 to 30 for the pubic louse. Eggs hatch in about a week.

Nymphs resemble miniature adults but are sexually immature. The first nymphal stage develops inside the egg. There are 3 molts over the 15 days to adulthood. Various published reports indicate that lice will live for 25 to 50 days, depending on the species. All lice live by sucking blood from the human host, every 3 to 6 hours. Once separated from their host, adult lice can survive without feeding for 2 to 10 days. The newborn head louse nymph, however, will die within 24 hours without a meal of human blood[22].

Pediculus humanus capitis

The adult head louse is 3 to 4 mm in length, gray-white in color, with three pairs of crab-like legs that are well adapted for grasping hairs. Because adult lice prefer to avoid light, they can move quickly along hairs and cannot readily be found on clinical examination. Reports differ somewhat in timing and total numbers, but during a lifespan of about one month, a female lays 7 to 10 eggs each day which hatch after 7 to 10 days. Nits are cemented to the hair shaft with chitin and are very difficult to remove (Figure 5). Initially fixed to the hairs close to the scalp, as the hair grows out, the nits move further out. Nits will not hatch at room temperature (i.e. away from the scalp) as they require a warm environment with a temperature of about 28°C (82°F) or higher, and humidity of 70%[23]. The translucent nit remains firmly attached to the hair shaft. The diagnosis is usually made by identification of nits, which can be seen by the naked eye. They must be distinguished from dried hair spray, dandruff and hair casts, which are not attached, but can be easily removed from the hair shaft, as well as piedra, which is also fixed to the hair.

Pediculus humanus corporis

The body louse is morphologically identical to the head louse, but is often a fraction larger. As do head lice, body lice feed on blood, sucked from the skin of the human host. Unlike head lice, however, the body louse fixes its nits to the fibers of clothing.

Pthirus pubis – Pubic (crab) lice

Pthirus pubis differs in morphology from the Pediculus species, being more crab-like in shape, with a more circular body, a first pair of legs and claws which are fine, and claws on the second and third pair of legs more widely spaced and capable of gripping two hairs. The adult louse may occasionally be found grasping two separate hairs in the pubic area. Elgart reports an interesting anecdote: the name Pthirus is actually an error and should be Phthirius. The incorrect spelling was officially registered with the International Committee of Zoological Nomenclature, and so it must remain! In spite of this, more articles in the literature use the non-official spelling (Phthirius) than the official spelling.

Epidemiology

Head lice are found worldwide. The highest incidence occurs in school-aged children, with girls more often affected than boys (although there is some difference of opinion in the literature) and without significant differences due to socioeconomic status, and although it is extremely uncommon in black Americans, it is commonly seen in black Africans. Hair length is not a factor.

Body lice are seen most commonly in times and areas of deprivation and crowding, such as among vagrants and the homeless who do not have access to bathing and laundry facilities, among the military when sanitation fails or is not available, and so historically was common to prisoner-of-war camps, concentration camps and foxholes. Today body lice are most often seen on the homeless in hospital emergency rooms, and the incidence of pediculosis corporis may be considered an index of poverty.

Crabs or pubic lice are also spread primarily by person to person contact, usually intimate contact, and may be considered a sexually transmitted disease. One third of patients with pubic lice may have other STDs.

Clinical features

The head louse is almost always confined to the scalp hair, although occasionally beard involvement may be seen. On the scalp, the occipital and postauricular regions will usually show the most involvement. An average host will have fewer than 20 adult lice, and fewer than 5% of patients will have more than 100 adult lice in the scalp. Head lice can survive away from the human host for about 3 days, and nits can survive for up to 10 days[22]. In one recent study of over 500 schoolchildren, the most common signs were pruritus, insect bite reaction and excoriations[24]. As with scabies, pruritus is thought to be caused by sensitization to the excreta or the body parts of the lice, and may take as long as 8 months to develop. Secondary infection with possible cervical adenopathy can accompany the infestation. Rarely, the blue macular bite reaction, macula cerulea, may be noted.

The disease is primarily spread from person to person by close physical contact but may be spread through fomites (for example combs, brushes, clothing, headgear, shared hats, earphones, bedding, upholstered furniture and rugs). There was one study that showed increased communicability of head lice among students in a school who shared lockers or coat hooks, and children who share a bed have been demonstrated to share their infection more than the siblings who sleep in a different bed.

The spread of lice, especially body lice, is encouraged by overcrowding. The body louse is the vector of *Rickettsia prowazekii*, the agent of epidemic typhus; *Bartonella quintana*, the agent of trench fever; and *Borrelia recurrentis*, the agent of relapsing fever, as well as salmonella. Body lice and their eggs are found predominantly on clothing and should be sought in the seams of clothes. *Pediculus humanus corporis* is rarely found on the skin, and the most common clinical finding is pyoderma with excoriation in covered areas, such as the groin, around the belt line and on the buttocks. Maculae ceruleae may be seen, but they are uncommon. The diagnosis is usually made when lice and nits are found in the interstices of the patient's garments, and in the emergency room, when a patient presents with a widespread pyoderma, alert personnel will shake out the clothes over the white paper covering the examining table, looking for lice.

The diagnosis of pubic lice is made by observation of the nit or adult louse. Here, too, maculae ceruleae may sometimes be found, but more often the nit or louse may be seen on the hair shaft. Crab lice prefer short hairs, most commonly the pubic area, but may be found on the eyelashes, eyebrows, beard, occipital scalp and body hair. Infestation of the eyelashes may be confused with other forms of blepharitis. They generally are asymptomatic for up to 30 days, but then they usually start to itch. The larvae attach to a single hair and take 7 to 8 days to mature, and then as adults they straddle two hairs. The finding of pubic lice on a child should alert one to the possibility of child abuse.

Treatment of pediculosis

The most effective pediculicides to date are those which contain permethrin (Nix®, a 1% creme rinse (Warner-Lambert Consumer Health Products, NJ), Elimite and Acticin, 5% creams) or malathion (Ovide®, Medicis, The Dermatology Company, AZ), the latter having just been approved by the FDA in the United States. Permethrin 1% creme rinse was compared to placebo in a double-blinded, randomized study with a third arm of the study including non-randomized, but investigator-blinded, treatment with 1% lindane shampoo. At 14 days after treatment, 97% of patients treated with permethrin were free of lice compared to 6% of placebo-treated patients and 43% of the lindane-treated group. Other studies have shown lindane to be somewhat more effective (98% treated with permethrin and 76% treated with lindane were louse-free 2 weeks after treatment, for example). Permethrin was 70% ovicidal compared to 14% of placebo and 45% for lindane[25]. Pyrethrum, a natural chrysanthemum derived product sold as A200 (Hogil Pharmaceutical Corp., NY), Pyrinate and RID (Pfizer, NY) also kills more rapidly than lindane and kills between about 68% and 77% of nits. Using these products strictly according to the instructions eliminates the need for nit removal after treatment, in spite of the 'zero nits policies' adopted by a number of school boards. One effective product for the removal of nits from the hair after pediculicide treatment is a creme rinse containing formic acid, Step 2 (Genderm, Lincolnshire, IL), that loosens the bond between the nit and hair. Another product marketed for this purpose is Clear Lice Egg Remover Gel (Care Technologies, Greenwich, CT), and alternatively, rinsing the scalp with a 50/50 vinegar/water mixture, and combing with a fine toothed comb may effectively remove many nits.

Lately there have been reports of a number of alternative treatments for resistant lice, referred to tongue-in-cheek as 'the head lice from hell'. These include petroleum jelly with or without occlusion. The theory is that the petroleum jelly blocks oxygen exchange. Likewise, mayonnaise (neither Light nor Miracle Whip), or olive oil have been recommended. Oral trimethoprim sulfa has been proposed, with a description that is quite graphic: 'Within 8–24 hours of administration of the TMP-sulfa, there is intense itching of the scalp and neck, and the lice could be seen crawling in these areas. Within the next 12–48 hours the lice migrated to the bed clothes and later died. During this period the lice could be seen falling off the hair in a very sluggish state'. Trimethoprim-sulfa works by killing symbiotic bacteria in the gut, and the lice starve to death; the nits produced are infertile because the bacteria are required for fertility. If nits are present, the patients should be re-treated in 10 days[26].

The treatment for pediculosis corporis is to bathe the patient with soap and water, and launder the garments in hot water. The use of an insecticide is unnecessary although this may help in wartime where bathing and changing clothes may not be feasible. In the hospital emergency room, office, or nursing home setting, it will suffice to take away the patient's clothes and give him or her clean clothes and a bath. Appropriate antibiotic therapy may be prescribed for the pyoderma.

In general, the treatment of pubic lice is simple. Lindane shampoo (applied for 5 minutes in the shower), lindane lotion (applied for 12 hours), pyrethrins such as A200, Pyrinate and RID (available without a prescription), 1% permethrin (Nix), and 0.5% malathion are all effective. Treatment is commonly repeated in 1 week to ten days[27]. Treatment failures are usually due to improper use of the medication rather than drug resistance, but failures are occasionally seen in male homosexuals and patients with large numbers of organisms. Infestations of the eyelashes may be treated with anticholinesterases such as neostigmine or physostigmine ophthalmic ointment, by applying a dab directly on the louse. Some authors recommend yellow oxide of mercury[28] or fluorescein, or even petrolatum applied twice daily for 7 to 10 days. The simplest technique for the treatment of eyelid lice is direct removal of the lice and nits. Sexual partners should be examined and simultaneously treated if infected, although it

would be reasonable to treat all household contacts to avoid reinfestation. Washing clothing and bed linen in hot water, or drying in a home clothes dryer, is adequate to eliminate the organisms. Persons with pubic lice should be examined for other sexually transmitted diseases.

CONCLUDING REMARKS

There is much wonderful material on the Internet, but some of it is wonderful misinformation. Because many patients, including both the geriatric population and their children and grandchildren, will access the net, the physician should be aware of the many web pages which highlight the side-effects of the proven treatments for pediculosis and scabies and recommend various unproven and alternative remedies, as well as the web pages which contain useful data. On a recent search for patient information concerning head lice, the majority of listings were from companies and organizations promoting alternative therapies such as herbal remedies, without regard to evidence-based data. The sites were, for the most part, very critical of the medically accepted treatments and exaggerated the toxicities of these regimens.

The National Pediculosis Association at http://www.headlice.org provides some very useful patient oriented information, albeit with a very strong bias against off label uses, and utilizes the web site to sell the LiceMeister® nit removal comb. The University of Oregon, at http://darkwing.uoregon.edu/~uoshc/scabiescrabslice.html has a very good handout. The CDC also has a web page of useful information at http://www.cdc.gov/ncidod/hip/abc/facts18.htm and http://www.cdc.gov/ncidod/dpd/parasites/headlice/default.htm. Considering the frequency with which pages appear and disappear on the world wide web, the Internet represents an excellent means of updating information for both the patient and the physician who is able to separate fact from fiction.

References

1. Sharbaugh R. Scabies: an itchy problem. *Home Care Provid* 1997;2:115–16
2. Barrett NJ, Morse DL. The resurgence of scabies. *Bur* 1993;3:R32–4
3. Degelau J. Scabies in long-term care facilities. *Infec Control Hosp Epidemiol* 1992;13:421–5
4. Burns DA. An outbreak of scabies in a residential home. *Br J Dermatol* 1987;117:359–61
5. Clayton R, Farrow S. Norwegian scabies following topical steroid therapy. *Postgrad Med J* 1975;51:657–9
6. Martin WE, Wheeler CE Jr. Diagnosis of human scabies by epidermal shave biopsy. *J Am Acad Dermatol* 1979;1:335–7
7. Woodley D, Saurat JH. The burrow ink test and the scabies mite. *J Am Acad Dermatol* 1981;4:715–22
8. Argenziano G, Fabbrocini G, Delfino M. Epiluminescence microscopy; a new approach to *in vivo* detection of *Sarcoptes scabiei*. *Arch Dermatol* 1997;133:751–3
9. Falk ES, Eide TJ. Histologic and clinical findings in human scabies. *Int J Dermatol* 1981;20:600–5
10. Franz TJ, Lehman PA, Franz SF, Guin JD. Comparative percutaneous absorption of lindane and permethrin. *Arch Dermatol* 1996;132:901–5
11. Olin BE, ed. *Drug Facts and Comparisons*. St Louis: Facts and Comparisons, Inc., 1998:3128–31
12. Schultz MW, Gomez M, Hansen RC, *et al.* Comparative study of 5% permethrin cream and 1% lindane lotion for the treatment of scabies. *Arch Dermatol* 1990;126:167–70
13. Glaziou P, Cartel JL, Alzieu P, *et al.* Comparison of ivermectin and benzyl benzoate for treatment of scabies. *Trop Med Parasitol* 1993;44:331–2
14. Kar SK, Mania J, Patnaik S. The use of ivermectin for scabies. *Natl Med J India* 1994;7:15–16
15. Sullivan JR. Successful use of ivermectin in the treatment of endemic scabies in a nursing home. *Australas J Dermatol* 1997;38:137–40
16. Barkwell R, Shields S. Deaths associated with ivermectin treatment of scabies [letter] [see comments]. *Lancet* 1997;349:1144–5
17. Bredal WP. Deaths associated with ivermectin for scabies [letter; comment]. *Lancet* 1997;350:216
18. Coyne PE, Addiss DG. Deaths associated with ivermectin for scabies [letter; comment]. *Lancet* 1997;350:215–16
19. Reintjes R, Hoek C. Deaths associated with ivermectin for scabies [letter; comment]. *Lancet* 1997;350:215; discussion 216
20. Diazgranados JA, Costa JL. Deaths after ivermectin treatment [letter]. *Lancet* 1997;349:1698
21. Elgart ML. Pediculosis. *Dermatol Clin* 1990;2:219–28
22. Witkowski JA, Parish LC. What's new in the management of lice. *Infect Med* 1997;14:28–96
23. Cheng TC. *General Parasitology*, 2nd ed. Orlando, Florida: Academic Press Inc., 1986:631–9. Quoted in Burkhardt CG. An assessment of topical and oral prescriptions and over-the-counter treatments for head lice. *J Am Acad Dermatol* 1998;38:979–82
24. Mumcuoglu KY. Clinical observations related to head lice infestation. *J Am Acad Dermatol* 1991;25(2 Pt 1):248–51
25. Taplin D. Permethrin 1% creme rinse for the treatment of *Pediculus humanus var capitis* infestation. *Pediatr Dermatol* 1986;3:344–8
26. Shashindran CH. Oral therapy of pediculosis capitis with Cotrimoxazole. *Br J Dermatol* 1978;98:699
27. Kalter DC, Sperber J, Rosen T, Matarasso S. *Arch Dermatol* 1987;123:1315–19
28. Ashkenazi I, Desatnik HR, Abraham FA. Yellow mercuric oxide: a treatment of choice for phthiriasis palpebrarum. *Br J Ophthalmol* 1991;75:356–8

Blistering diseases in the elderly 8

N. Sami and A. R. Ahmed

INTRODUCTION

Blistering diseases are rare in the elderly; however, since the elderly population is increasing, the frequency and incidence are likely to increase also. Although they are rare, many can have a serious or even fatal outcome. There is a vast number of skin and systemic diseases in which blisters may be present, either as a primary manifestation or as part of a multisystemic disease. In this chapter blistering diseases with a known autoimmune mechanism of pathogenesis are discussed. The intent of the authors is not to be all inclusive but to focus on the more common blistering diseases. The pathogenesis, clinical manifestations, histology and basis for treatment are discussed. The reader is advised that the therapy of such patients is best delivered in close consultation and co-operation with a dermatologist. The diseases discussed in this chapter are as follows: pemphigus vulgaris, bullous pemphigoid, mucous membrane pemphigoid, epidermolysis bullosa acquisita, dermatitis herpetiformis, porphyria cutanea tarda and linear IgA dermatosis. Bullous disease of the comatose, subcorneal pustular dermatosis and transient acantholytic dermatosis are briefly mentioned to facilitate differential diagnosis.

PEMPHIGUS

Pemphigus is a rare blistering disease that affects the skin and the mucous membranes; it has many variants, the vulgaris form being most common[1]. Less common ones include vegetans, foliaceus, erythematosus, drug-induced and fogo selvagem[2,3]. Pemphigus vulgaris affects both genders equally, with the majority age of presentation being 50–60 years old[3]. The worldwide incidence is very low, with a higher incidence seen in Ashkenazi Jews[1].

Clinical features

Blisters are flaccid and easily rupture, resulting in large painful erosions[3]. These lesions can heal or spread further at their periphery. Healing usually occurs without scarring and is often accompanied by post-inflammatory hyperpigmentation[4]. A Nikolsky's sign can be exhibited by applying pressure on the periphery of the bullae and extending these lesions laterally[3]. Initial presentation in the majority of patients with pemphigus vulgaris is in the oral cavity (Figures 1 and 2)[4]. In contrast patients with pemphigus foliaceus initially present with lesions affecting the skin of the face, scalp and trunk (Figures 3 and 4)[5]. Other mucosal areas commonly affected by pemphigus vulgaris include the larynx, pharynx, esophagus, anus and genitalia[1,3]. When the skin is involved in pemphigus vulgaris it usually presents on the face, trunk, back, breast, groin and axillae (Figures 3 and 4)[1]. Pemphigus vulgaris must be differentiated from paraneoplastic pemphigus, which is not a true pemphigus but a complex of symptoms with a clinical heterogeneous phenotype with some lesions that resemble pemphigus vulgaris and erythema multiforme. It affects the skin and mucosal tissues, and is associated with tumors such as lymphomas, chronic lymphocytic leukemia and bronchogenic carcinoma.

Drug-induced pemphigus tends to present initially as an urticarial rash which normally results eventually in pemphigus foliaceus, but occasionally as pemphigus vulgaris[7]. The

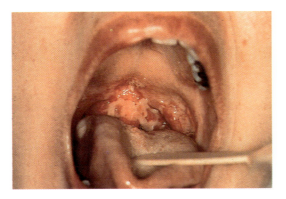

Figure 1 Pemphigus vulgaris: this patient presented initially with erosive lesions on the soft palate and buccal mucosa. Figure reproduced with permission from Scott VE, Ahmed AR. The blistering diseases. *Med Clin North Am* 1998;82:1239–83

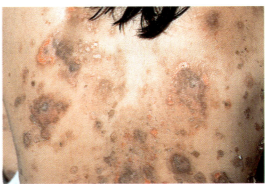

Figure 3 Pemphigus foliaceus: confluent erosions on the back

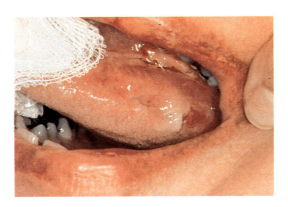

Figure 2 Pemphigus vulgaris: erosive lesions on the lateral side of the tongue and at the junction of the tongue and sublingual mucosa. Figure reproduced with permission from Scott VE, Ahmed AR. The blistering diseases. *Med Clin North Am* 1998;82:1239–83

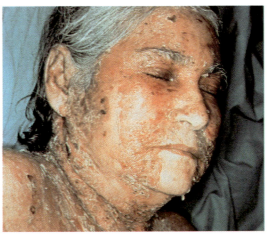

Figure 4 Pemphigus foliaceus: erosions, intact vesicles and significant adherent crusting on the scalp, face and neck in an elderly woman

typical pemphigus lesions can develop months later and may not resolve despite termination of drug use[2,3]. Drugs commonly seen to cause pemphigoid lesions include penicillamine, captopril, penicillin, ceftazidime, rifampin, β-blockers, progesterone, heroin and pyrazalone compounds[3,7,8].

Pemphigus vegetans is a rare form of pemphigus known to affect the tongue in what is known as cereberiform tongue[1,9]. It is further classified as the Neumann and Hallopeau subtypes[9]. The Hallopeau subtype presents with pustules affecting the intertriginous areas[1,2], while the Neumman subtype presents with ruptured bullae with pustules seen on the periphery of the lesions[1,4], which can later form hyperkeratotic vegetating lesions[4].

Pathology

Pemphigus is characterized by acantholysis[10]. Autoantibodies are produced against an intercellular substance (ICS) which binds epidermal cells through desmosomes. These anti-ICS antibodies bind to the antigen on the

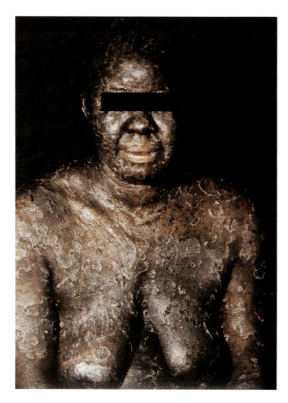

Figure 5   Bullous pemphigoid in a generalized distribution in an African-American patient

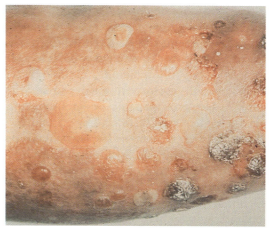

Figure 6   Bullous pemphigoid: vesicles and large tense bullae are seen with adherent crusting from the drying of blister fluid

Differential diagnosis

The differential diagnosis of pemphigus includes bullous pemphigoid, mucous membrane pemphigoid, epidermolysis bullous acquisita, porphyria cutanea tarda, erosive lichen planus, Behçet's disease, acute herpetic stomatitis, necrotizing gingivostomatitis and hand-foot-and-mouth disease[1].

Treatment

Owing to the rate of morbidity and mortality, pemphigus lesions should be treated aggressively with systemic as well as topical treatments. However, treatment should be individualized depending on the extent of the disease. The most commonly used drugs to treat pemphigus are corticosteroids and immunosuppressives. Patients with localized pemphigus are initially treated with topical and intralesional corticosteroids[3,4,12,13]. However, dapsone and tetracycline, or antimalarials, can be added for adequate treatment[7]. Systemic corticosteroids should be used for generalized pemphigus and for refractory localized disease[1,6,14]. Patients respond well to 20–40 mg/day in moderate disease and 60 mg/day in severe disease[13]. Since systemic corticosteroids are associated

epidermis, activating enzymes responsible for the conversion of plasminogen to plasmin. Plasmin further causes breakdown of the ICS leading to acantholysis and, therefore, blister formation[10,11]. On histology, acantholysis within the epidermis is the hallmark of pemphigus, with characteristic intra-epidermal vesicle formation. In pemphigus vulgaris and vegetans the vesicle is suprabasilar.

Pemphigus foliaceus and erythematosus are characterized by subcorneal vesicle formation. On direct immunofluorescence (DIF), a homogeneous intercellular deposition of IgG and C3 is seen in affected and surrounding areas[1]. The sera of pemphigus vulgaris and pemphigus foliaceus patients contain an antibody that binds to the ICS of the substrate on which it is tested. In a majority of patients the titer of the autoantibody parallels disease activity and severity.

with increased side-effects, especially in the elderly, concomitant use of other immuno-suppressive agents can help reduce the doses of corticosteroids. These agents include aza-thioprine, cyclophosphamide, methotrexate, chlorambucil, cyclosporine, dapsone and gold[2,12]. However, patients on methotrexate have a higher rate of infections[1,15], and the most effective combinations are corticosteroids with azathioprine or cyclophosphamide[12]. Plasmapharesis should only be used when all other therapies have failed, and may require simultaneous cyclophosphamide to reduce rebound autoantibody synthesis[1]. Alternative strategies of treatment for patients include intravenous immunoglobulin[12].

Prognosis

The prognosis of pemphigus varies with its subtype along with several other factors. Pem-phigus foliaceus and erythematosus have a better prognosis compared to vulgaris and vegetans. However the use of corticosteroid therapy has significantly reduced mortality to about 10% in PV[3,13]. Factors which can predict a poor clinical course include age of onset, disease progression and response to cortico-steroid treatment[13].

BULLOUS PEMPHIGOID

Bullous pemphigoid is an autoimmune blis-tering disease of the elderly which occurs most frequently in individuals over 70 years of age[16]. It occurs in all races worldwide and mainly affects the skin[17–19].

Clinical features

The initial symptoms can mimic a benign pruritic eczematous dermatitis or an urticarial rash which fails to disappear in 24 to 48 hours and can progress to tense bullae and blisters within weeks to months (Figure 5)[4]. These blisters may be single or multiple and present on erythematous or normal appearing skin (Figure 6)[20,21]. The fluid in these bullae can be hemorrhagic or clear. The bullae range in diameter from 0.5 to 7 cm, which can help to differentiate them clinically from pemphi-gus[4]. Once ruptured, bullae heal leaving post-inflammatory pigmentary changes[4].

In addition, bullous and urticarial pem-phigoid presentations include vesicular, papular, vegetating, seborrheic and erythro-dermic[22,23]. The papular or nodular variety, also known as pemphigoid nodularis, presents initially as hyperkeratotic nodules that later progress to bullae over several years[23,24]. The erythrodermic variant is a generalized erythema occurring with bullae while the vesic-ular variant presents as heterogeneous vesic-ulobullous lesions. A bullous pemphigoid-like disease has been associated with some drugs, including furosemide and phenacetin[18,22]. Lichen planus and psoriasis have been asso-ciated with bullous pemphigoid, as have autoimmune diseases such as diabetes, perni-cious anemia, rheumatoid arthritis and multiple sclerosis. Bullous pemphigoid has been seen in malignancies of the gastro-intestinal tract, urinary tract, lymphoreticular system, pancreas, genitalia, breast, lung and skin[18,25]. However, no causal relationship has been established.

Differential diagnosis

Bullous pemphigoid should always be consid-ered in patients presenting with large tense pruritic bullae. However, other diseases to be considered in the differential diagnosis include pemphigus vulgaris, dermatitis her-petiformis, epidermolysis bullosa acquista and erythema multiforme.

Pathology

Bullous pemphigoid is characterized by a subepidermal vesicle or bullae of the underly-ing dermis. These lesions may be poor or rich in inflammatory infiltrate. The infiltrate may be fixed or predominantly polymor-phonuclear and eosinophilic in nature. The diagnosis of bullous pemphigoid is confirmed by the presence of immunoglobulins, most frequently IgG, and complement at the basement membrane of the perilesional skin. Anti-basement membrane antibodies are determined in the sera of 70–80% of patients with bullous pemphigoid[22]. The salt-split skin technique shows IgG bound to the intact roof side of the split and this differentiates it from epidermolysis bullosa acquisita[20].

Prognosis

The clinical course of bullous pemphigoid is unpredictable. It can be self-limiting with a spontaneous early remission or can have a long protracted chronic course. However, it has a relatively better prognosis than other blistering diseases like pemphigus vulgaris, mucous membrane pemphigoid and epidermolysis bullosa. Factors that have an impact on prognosis include age and extent of disease. Bullous pemphigoid can be fatal if left untreated or inappropriately treated, with mortality ranging from 20 to 30%[26–28].

Treatment

Bullous pemphigoid can be treated with both local and systemic therapies, the drugs of choice used to treat it being systemic corticosteroids[18]. Initially, prednisone should be given in divided doses in the acute phase of the disease. The daily dose of prednisone should be prescribed according to the severity of the disease, with mild cases receiving 20 mg, moderate cases 40–60 mg and severe cases 60–80 mg. Only in very rare instances have patients needed doses of 100 mg or more. However, it is important to note that the elderly are more prone to the diverse side-effects of corticosteroids. Therefore other therapies can be adopted to minimize the dosage of steroids. These include co-administration of immunosuppressive agents with steroids, for example sulfapyridine, azathioprine and methotrexate[18]. Of these, methotrexate is best tolerated in the elderly and is best administered as 2.5–5.0 mg per day for 2–3 days in a week[29,30]. Azathioprine is another frequently used immunosuppressive agent, with effective dosages of 1–1.5 mg/kg/day[31]. Because of its

suppression of the bone marrow, complete blood counts should be monitored weekly for the first 2 months, every other week for the next 2 months, and monthly thereafter. Other immunosuppressives which have been successfully used include chlorambucil and cyclosporine[22,32].

Dapsone or antibiotics like tetracycline and erythromycin can be given to patients in whom corticosteroids are contraindicated. Owing to dapsone's bone marrow suppression, hepatotoxicity and hemolytic side-effects, it is recommended that patients initiate low dose therapy with 25 mg daily for 3 days followed by subsequent incremental increases of 25 mg twice daily for 3 days, 25 mg three times daily for 7 days, 50 mg twice daily for 3 days, finally reaching a daily therapeutic dose of 150–200 mg[33–35].

Plasmapharesis should be used in bullous pemphigoid when it is severe, has failed to respond to other chemotherapeutic agents and as a last resort. This is because the rate of recurrence and incidence of side-effects of plasmapharesis is similar to that of other systemic therapies[36].

The use of intralesional corticosteroids is not very common. However, this therapy can prove to be an alternative mode of treatment in patients with localized disease or in whom systemic corticosteroids are contraindicated. Most lesions respond to intralesional injections of triamcinolone acetonide at dilutions of 5 mg/ml. In more resistant lesions dilutions of 7.5–10 mg/ml have been effective[37].

It is important to note that among the highest causes of mortality in bullous pemphigoid has been infection. If adequate topical care is not given, the fluid in the blisters can prove to be a good culture medium for bacteria. Therefore aggressive topical management and maintenance of hygiene are important. Potassium manganate VII (potassium permanganate) or aluminum subacetate solutions in a Hubbard tank or bathtub can prove to be beneficial. Blisters should only be dressed with one layer of Kerlix gauze over the lesions. If there is a suspicion of infection in the blisters, a culture should be taken and appropriate antibiotics should be given once the offending organism is identified[37].

MUCOUS MEMBRANE PEMPHIGOID

Mucous membrane pemphigoid (MMP), also known as cicatricial pemphigoid, is an autoimmune subepidermal blistering disease that primarily affects the elderly[38]. This disease is 1.5 times more prevalent in women than men, with an average age of onset of 62 years and no racial predilection[38,39]. It mainly affects the mucous membranes[38,39].

Clinical features

All stratified squamous epithelium can be involved in mucous membrane pemphigoid, that is the mucosa of the oral cavity, nose, nasopharynx, pharynx, esophagus, larynx, trachea, eye, pelvis, vagina and anal canal. The reported incidence is often biased by the specialty of the investigator. The eye is involved in 65% of MMP patients and the oral cavity in about 85%[2,39]. The frequency of involvement of other mucosae has been reviewed by Ahmed, Kurgis and Rogers[39]. Symptoms are dependent on the site(s) of involvement. Conjunctival lesions initially manifest as irritation, burning, increased lacrimation, photophobia and dryness of the eyes. These symptoms are initially unilateral but can become bilateral within two years[39]. Lesions in the oral cavity may accompany those at all anatomic sites, but are frequently seen as a 'desquamative gingivitis'. Nasal involvement presents with discharge and epistaxis while pharyngeal and esophageal involvement can present as dysphagia[2,39]. Lesions involving the mucosal membranes of the larynx and trachea can present as hoarseness, aphonia and even dyspnea[2,39]. As the disease progresses, stenosis occurs owing to submucosal fibrosis, especially in the pharynx, esophagus, larynx and vagina[2,40]. Blindness occurs because of contouring shrinkage ectropion and corneal ulceration. Skin involvement can occur on the scalp, face, head and neck,

trunk and extremities[39,41]. This is known as the Brunsting–Perry variety and it usually heals with atrophic scars. Disease limited to the oral cavity may present with problems of nutrition. Involvement of the eyes, pharynx, larynx and esophagus carry an unpredictable prognosis.

PATHOLOGY

The diagnosis can be confirmed on routine histology by the presence of submucosal vesicles or with an infiltrate composed of lymphocytes, eosinophils and neutrophils in the submucosa[42]. Upper papillary submucosal fibrosis can be seen in many lesions[42]. As with bullous pemphigoid, direct immunofluorescence shows a homogeneous linear complement deposition of IgG and C3 on the basement membrane[22]. There have been few reports of IgA and IgM deposition[22]. IgG circulating anti-basement membrane antibody titers have been demonstrated in up to 20–30% of MMP patients[39]. Salt-split-skin techniques have shown that anti-basement membrane antibodies can bind to the roof of the blister side of the basement membrane[39].

Treatment

Initial treatment of MMP is usually with local therapies and systemic dapsone. Systemic corticosteroids and adjuvant immunosuppressives like cyclophosphamide are given if lesions are progressive or fail to respond to dapsone[40]. Cyclophosphamide is given at a dose of 0.5–1.5 mg/kg/day[43]. However, patients should be warned about the side-effects of this chemotherapeutic agent, like alopecia and hemorrhagic cystitis[43]. Aggressive treatment is recommended in ocular MMP. Prophylactic or reconstructive surgery may be necessary where lesions have progressed to stenosis and threaten life or can cause physiologic dysfunction.

EPIDERMOLYSIS BULLOSA ACQUISITA

Epidermolysis bullosa acquisita (EBA) is a subepidermal blistering disease which can

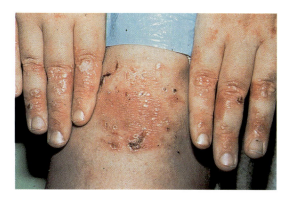

Figure 7   Epidermolysis bullosa acquisita: patient with milia and atrophic scarring on dorsum of fingers and knee

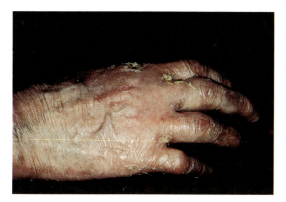

Figure 8   Epidermolysis bullosa acquisita: multiple tense blisters on the dorsa of the hand

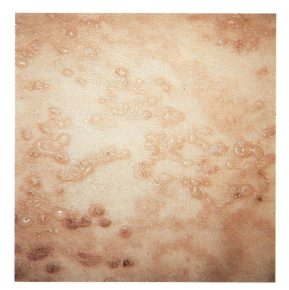

Figure 9   Dermatitis herpetiformis: vesicles, papules and small bullae on the thigh of a patient

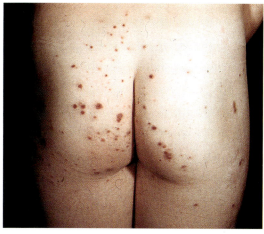

Figure 10   Dermatitis herpetiformis: multiple papular and vesicular lesions on the sacrum and buttocks

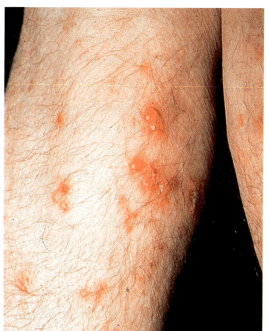

Figure 11   Linear IgA dermatosis: multiple intact vesicles on an erythematous base on the lower legs

resemble other blistering diseases like bullous pemphigoid and cicatricial pemphigoid in its clinical presentation. It affects the elderly, with equal prevalence in both sexes and all races and can affect those with no family history of bullous disease[44].

Clinical features

EBA lesions are characterized by skin fragility, tense blisters and erosions in areas of easy bruisibility or trauma. The blisters contain serous or hemorrhagic fluid. These lesions often heal forming milia and atrophic scars (Figure 7)[22]. EBA is most commonly seen on extensor surfaces, especially over the hands and feet (Figure 8)[4], where nail involvement presents as dystrophic nail plates[2]. EBA has been reported to affect mucous membranes of the eyes, oral cavity, larynx, esophagus and urogenital tract[44]. The scalp can also be involved, healing with scarring alopecia[2]. There have been reported associations with other skin disorders such as psoriasis as well as systemic diseases such as collagen vascular disease, inflammatory bowel disease, thyroiditis, infections and malignancies, notably multiple myeloma[2,45–47].

Pathology

The blister is subepidermal in location and in some patients is accompanied by an inflammatory infiltrate, though in others there is no infiltrate at all. A linear deposition of immunoglobulins (IgG) and complement (C3) is seen on the basement membrane on direct immunofluorescence[22,48]. The IgG deposits on the lower part of the lamina densa of the basement membranes on immune electron microscopy[48]. On salt-split-skin techniques, EBA sera bind to the dermal side of the split[48].

Differential diagnosis

The differential diagnosis of EBA includes bullous pemphigus, MMP and porphyria cutanea tarda. A clinical history of trauma-induced bullae which heal with scarring is not very common in the other entities. Porphyria cutanea tarda, which can also present with bullae that heal with scarring and milia, can be differentiated with urine porphyrin studies[37].

Treatment

Differentiating EBA from other blistering diseases becomes important for determining treatment options. Drugs which have been used to treat EBA include steroids, dapsone, gold, phenytoin, colchicine and vitamin E, but immunosuppressants like cyclophosphamide, cyclosporine and azathioprine have provided either no improvement or minimal temporary improvement[44,49]. However, most of these drugs provoke intolerant and potentially catastrophic and fatal side-effects, especially in the elderly. Plasmapharesis and extracorporeal photochemotherapy show some success[44,50]. The recent use of intravenous immunoglobulins has shown significant promise and cause for optimism. Because of the lack of successful treatment options available, it is important to consider other supportive measures which can improve healing. These include encouraging good nutrition, treating infections with local and systemic antibiotics and protecting the skin from subsequent trauma.

Prognosis

This blistering disease tends to run a chronic course in most patients, with very few having spontaneous improvement and many having recurrent flares after temporary remission[2]. The disease can run a severe course from the primary blistering lesions and atrophic scarring[44]. Morbidity is determined by the area and extent of involvement of the skin and mucosa[44] and lesions involving the oral cavity, esophagus, and lower extremities can be severely disabling.

DERMATITIS HERPETIFORMIS

Dermatitis herpetiformis is a blistering disease rarely reported in the elderly. This autoimmune disease has a slightly higher male predominance and occurs in people with European descent[51]. Patients affected by dermatitis herpetiformis also have a higher incidence of such autoimmune diseases as diabetes mellitus, thyroiditis and pernicious anemia, and small bowel lymphoma and atrophic gastritis have been reported to accompany the disease[2,4,52,53]. The majority of dermatitis herpetiformis patients have small bowel pathology identical to that of celiac disease[52,53]. These lesions are scattered, asymptomatic, microscopic and of no clinical consequence to the patient.

Clinical features

Patients with dermatitis herpetiformis can experience localized symptoms of stinging, itching, or burning almost 12 hours prior to the eruption of the lesions[52]. Pruritus which is generalized, severe, extreme and disproportionate to the skin lesions is prevalent and can be one of the hallmarks of the disease. Lesions are vesicles, papules, urticaria, or small bullae (Figure 9)[4]. They can be symmetrically distributed, often grouped together or scattered on the face, facial hairline, shoulders, knees, buttocks, sacral areas and extensor surfaces of the forearms (Figure 10)[51,52].

Pathology

Routine histology shows vesicles in the dermal papillae with an inflammatory infiltrate made up of eosinophils and neutrophils[51], called eosinophilic abscess. Direct immunofluorescence shows characteristic granular deposition of IgA at the tips of the dermal papillae. Sera contain an IgA antibody to endomyosium[51,54], which may correlate with disease activity and severity.

Treatment

The treatment of dermatitis herpetiformis is two-fold. First, patients should initially be treated with dapsone unless this is contraindicated[51,55], a major contraindication being glucose-6-phosphate deficiency. However, cimetidine can be prescribed with dapsone to help reduce the hemolytic side-effects[55]. The starting dose should be 100 mg/day with a maintenance dose of 25–200 mg/day[53,55]. Other effective combinations include tetracycline

and nicotinamide[56]. The second treatment modality is elimination of gluten from the diet. After a prolonged gluten-free diet patients can eventually be weaned off all systemic drugs, including dapsone, and recurrence of the disease can be prevented[57,58].

Prognosis

Dermatitis herpetiformis is a chronic disease characterized by relapses and remissions. A gluten-free diet can significantly ameliorate the disease and provide a high quality of life[58].

PORPHYRIA CUTANEA TARDA

Porphyria cutanea tarda (PCT) is an uncommon metabolic disease associated with blisters. The incidence of PCT in the general population is one in twenty-five thousand[59]. PCT patients have dysfunctional urogen decarboxylase, an enzyme involved in heme synthesis leading to an increase in porphyrin levels and iron overload in the body[60]. Factors known to exacerbate PCT include alcohol, estrogen and polychlorinated cyclic hydrocarbons[61].

Clinical features

The majority of PCT patients present with serous or hemorrhagic vesicles or bullae on areas of the body that have been exposed to the sun, including the face and dorsa of the hands and forearms, which heal with scarring[59,62]. The healing may take several weeks and result in post-inflammatory hyperpigmentation, milia and atrophic scars. Other cutaneous manifestations of PCT include hypertrichosis on the forehead and face, hypopigmented yellowish plaques, scarring alopecia and onycholysis[62,63].

The diagnosis of porphyria should be made after screening urine and blood for porphyrins[64]. The total amount of porphyrins excreted in 24 hours in usually greater than 1000 micrograms[64]. The urine is examined with a Wood's lamp and exhibits a reddish-pink color if PCT is present. Elevated levels of iron, ferritin and transaminases in serum are also seen in PCT[62,63].

Pathology

On histology, a subepidermal blister with minimal or little inflammatory infiltrate in the dermis is observed[65]. The capillary walls in the papillary dermis are thickened and usually stain positive with periodic acid–Schiff reagent (PAS)[65]. Direct immunofluorescence of perilesional skin shows C3, IgG and IgM in the capillary walls and dermo-epidermal junction[65].

Differential diagnosis

The differential diagnosis of PCT includes pseudoporphyria, variegate porphyria (VP) and epidermolysis bullosa acquisita. Pseudo-porphyria is a condition associated with patients being treated with nalidixic acid, tetracycline and furosemide or patients on hemodialysis for chronic renal failure. Patients with pseudoporphyria have cutaneous manifestations similar to those of PCT but normal porphyrin levels[66].

Treatment

The treatment of PCT is two-fold. First, factors known to exacerbate PCT, if present, should be avoided[62]. Secondly, patients should undergo weekly or bi-weekly phlebotomy until a hemoglobin count of 10 g/dl or serum iron concentration of 50 μg/dl is achieved[62]. Clinical improvement of lesions is usually observed 3–6 months later[62]. Patients for whom phlebotomy is contraindicated have been successfully treated with chloroquine and hydroxychloroquine[67]. Remissions with the above treatment have been shown to last an average of 31 months[63].

LINEAR IGA DERMATOSIS

Linear IgA dermatosis (LAD) is one of the less common subepidermal blistering diseases found in the elderly and affects women more often than men[2]. A LAD-like clinical picture has been reported in some patients being treated with vancomycin, lithium carbonate, diclofenac and glibenclamide or patients with lymphoma[68].

Clinical features

LAD affects the skin more than the mucous membranes of the body, with clinical features of multiple blistering diseases resembling bullous pemphigoid, dermatitis herpetiformis and bullous erosions[40,68]. The lesion can present as an urticarial plaque with surrounding vesicles (Figure 11)[2,68]. The distribution of these vesicles is characterized as being like a string of pearls. In some LAD patients mucosal lesions typically present as either single or multiple.

Pathology

On histology LAD resembles dermatitis herpetiformis with subepidermal vesicles and neutrophils in the dermal papillary tips and vacuolization of the basal cells[2,51,68]. The diagnosis can be confirmed by direct immunofluorescence with a homogeneous linear deposition of IgA only seen along the dermal-epidermal junction[2,51,68]. Indirect immunofluorescence is usually negative. When immunoblot assay is available, LAD sera can be demonstrated binding to 97 kDa protein in epidermal extracts, presumably a hemidesmosome protein.

Treatment

The mainstay of treatment of LAD is dapsone and sulfapyridine[2]. Other treatment options are available but have had limited success, including systemic corticosteroids and a combination of nicotinamide and tetracycline[69]. Occasionally LAD patients go into spontaneous remission within two years of onset[2,69], though most patients run a chronic clinical course[2].

BULLOUS DISEASE OF THE COMATOSE

Bullous disease of the comatose (coma bullae) is a rare blistering disease found in as many as 6.5% of unconscious patients[70]. This disease was first described in 1812 in soldiers of Napoleon's army intoxicated with carbon monoxide[71] and it was later associated in patients with barbiturate intoxication[72]. Various theories have been proposed as to the etiology of bullae appearing in comatose patients. These include trauma, localized hypoxia, eccrine fatigue from excessive sweating and drug build up in the eccrine glands[73]. Opiates, tricyclic antidepressants, meprobamate, glutethimide and methaqualone are a few of the drugs associated with coma bullae. In the comatose, pathologic conditions associated with coma bullae are diabetic ketoacidosis, CNS lesions (trauma, stroke, tumors and infection), and hypercalcemia from hyperparathyroidism[73–76]. A similar clinical profile has been observed in patients undergoing dialysis for chronic renal failure.

Clinical features

The bullae usually present within 12 to 24 hours after loss of consciousness over pressure areas of the body like bony prominences and the inner knees[70]. The initial presentation is a dusky red or echymotic macular lesion, which is unilateral and linear[70]. These macules can progress to form tense hemorrhagic bullae which can undergo necrosis and penetrate deeper into fat and muscle if not managed properly[71]. Mucosal lesions are invariably absent.

Pathology

Histologically, subepidermal bullae with no or minimal subepidermal inflammation in eccrine gland necrosis may be present[77]. On direct immunofluorescence, IgM and C3 deposition is seen in the upper dermal vessel in some patients[77].

Treatment

The treatment of bullae in the comatose is mainly supportive topical care by preventing superinfections and relieving any underlying external pressure thought to be the etiology of the lesions. Most lesions heal without scarring in 2–3 weeks[72].

SUBCORNEAL PUSTULAR DERMATOSIS

Subcorneal pustular dermatosis (SCPD), also known as Sneddon–Wilkinson syndrome, is a benign bullous disease which affects four times as many women as men[78]. The lesions present as crops of sterile pustular eruptions in an annular pattern that have a serpiginous outline. These lesions are most commonly seen in the cornea, groin, axillary and inframammary areas, and extensor aspects of upper and lower limbs[78]. On histology, subcorneal bullae are seen with an inflammatory infiltrate made mainly of neutrophils. SCPD is treated systemically with dapsone at 50–150 mg daily. Sulfapyridine and high dose systemic corticosteroids can be used as an alternative. The disease runs a chronic recurrent course lasting up to eight years[78].

TRANSIENT ACANTHOLYTIC DERMATOSIS

Transient acantholytic dermatosis (TAD), also known as Grover's disease, presents frequently in people from 40 to 60 years of age with a history of extensive actinic damage[79]. There seems to be some association between TAD and blockage of the sweat glands. The lesions present as pruritic vesicles on the neck, chest and back, which crust and heal without scarring. Histologically, the vesicle is intra-epidermal with acantholysis and dyskeratosis[80]. The lesions are usually self-limiting and usually last for from several months to a year. Local systemic steroids have been shown to be effective in their treatment, and patients who keep exposure to heat and the sun to a minimum may recover more quickly[81].

References

1. Becker BA, Gaspari AA. Pemphigus vulgaris and vegetans: bullous diseases. *Dermatol Clin* 1993;11:429–52

2. Fine JD. Bullous diseases. In Moschella SL, Hurley HJ, eds. *Dermatology*, 3rd edn. Philadelphia: WB Saunders, 1992:656–81

3. Stanely JR. Pemphigus. In Fitzpatrick TB, Eisen AZ, Wolff K, *et al.*, eds. *Dermatology in General Medicine*, 5th edn. New York: McGraw-Hill, 1999:654–66

4. Pye RJ. Bullous eruptions. In Champion RH, Burton JL, Ebling FJR, eds. *Rook/Wilkinson/Ebling Textbook of Dermatology*, 5th edn. Oxford: Blackwell Scientific, 1992:1638–65

5. Lee CW, Ro YS. Pemphigus developed on preexisting dermatoses. *J Dermatol* 1994;21:213–15

6. Mutasim DF, Pelc NJ, Anhalt GJ. Paraneoplastic pemphigus: bullous diseases. *Dermatol Clin* 1993;11:473–81

7. Kuechle MK, Hutton KP, Muller SA. Angiotensin-converting enzyme inhibitor induced pemphigus: three case reports and literature review. *Mayo Clin Proc* 1994;69:1166–71

8. Pellicano R, Janmantuono M, Lomuto M. Pemphigus erythematosus induced by ceftazidime. *Int J Dermatol* 1993;32:675–6

9. Sawai T, Kitazawa K, Danno K, *et al.* Pemphigus vegetans with esophageal involvement: successful treatment with minocycline and nicotinamide. Correspondence. *Br J Dermatol* 1995;132:668–70

10. Mobini N, Ahmed AR. Bullous diseases. In McDonald CJ, ed. *Immunomudulatory and Cytotoxic Agents in Dermatology*. New York: Marcel Dekker, 1996:70–85

11. Sams WM Jr, Gammon WR. Mechanism of lesion production in pemphigus and pemphigoid. *J Am Acad Dermatol* 1982;6:431–52

12. Huilgol SC, Black MM. Management of immunobullous disorders. II. Pemphigus. (Review article). *Clin Exp Dermatol* 1995;20:283–93

13. Tehranchi-Nia Z, Qureshi TA, Ahmed AR. Pemphigus vulgaris in older adults. *J Am Geriatr Soc* 1998;46:92–4

14. Deloach-Banta LJ, Tenaro LJ. Superficial erosions with some oozing and marked crusting: pemphigus erythematosus. *Arch Dermatol* 1993;129:633, 636–7

15. Carson PJ, Hameed A, Ahmed AR. Influence of treatment on the clinical course of pemphigus vulgaris. *J Am Acad Dermatol* 1996;34:645–52

16. Rook AJ, Waddington E. Pemphigus and pemphigoid. *Br J Dermatol* 1953;65:425–31

17. Lim CC, MacDonald RH, Rook AJ. Pemphigoid eruptions in the elderly. *Trans St John's Hosp Dermatol Soc Lond* 1968;54:148–51

18. Koch CA, Mazzaferri EL, Larry LA, *et al.* Bullous pemphigoid after treatment with furosemide: continuing medical education. *Cutis* 1996;58:340–4

19. Nousari HC, Anhalt GJ. Pemphigus and bullous pemphigoid. *Lancet* 1997;354:667–72

20. Stanley JR. Bullous pemphigoid, cicatricial pemphigoid, and chronic bullous disease of childhood. In Fitzpatrick TB, Eisen AZ, Wolff K, *et al.*, eds. *Dermatology in General Medicine*, 4th edn. New York: McGraw-Hill, 1993:615–26

21. Korman NJ. Bullous pemphigoid. The latest in diagnosis, prognosis and therapy. *Arch Dermatol* 1998;134:1137–41

22. Cliff S, Holden CA. Pemphigoid nodularis: a report of three cases and review of literature. *Br J Dermatol* 1997;136:398–401

23. Bourke JF, Berth-Jonees J, Gawkrodger DJ, *et al.* Pemphigoid nodularis: a report of two cases. *Clin Exp Dermatol* 1994;19:496–9

24. Korman NJ. Bullous pemphigoid: bullous diseases. *Dermatol Clin* 1993;11:483–98

25. Kirtchig G, Walkden VM, Venning VA, *et al.* Bullous pemphigoid and multiple sclerosis: a report of three cases and review of the literature. *Clin Exp Dermatol* 1995;20:449–53

26. Roujeau JC, Lok C, Batuji-Garin G, *et al.* High risk of death in elderly patients with extensive bullous pemphigoid. *Arch Dermatol* 1998;134:465–9

27. Savin JA. The events leading to the death of patients in pemphigus and bullous pemphigoid. *Br J Dermatol* 1979;101:521–34

28. Mondino BJ, Brown SI. Ocular cicatricial pemphigoid. *Ophthalmology* 1981;88:95–100

29. Downham TF, Chapel TA. Bullous pemphigoid: therapy in patients with and without diabetes mellitus. *Arch Dermatol* 1978;114:1639–42

30. Paul MA, Jorizzo JL, Fleischer AB Jr, *et al.* Low dose methotrexate treatment in the elderly patient with bullous pemphigoid. *J Am Acad Dermatol* 1994;31:620–5

31. Ahmed AR, Maize JC, Provost TT. Bullous pemphigoid: clinical and immunologic follow up after successful therapy. *Arch Dermatol* 1977;113:1043–6

32. Thiovolet J, Barthelemy H, Rogot-Muller G, *et al.* Effects of cyclosporin in bullous pemphigoid and pemphigus. *Lancet* 1985;1:334–5

33. Piamphongsant T. Dapsone for the treatment of bullous pemphigoid. *Asian Pacific J Allergy Immunol* 1983;1:19–21

34. Roger RS, Seehafer JR, Perry HO. Treatment of cicatricial pemphigoid with dapsone. *J Am Acad Dermatol* 1982;6:215–23

35. Lang PJ. Sulfones and sulfonamides in dermatology today. *J Am Acad Dermatol* 1979;1: 479–92

36. Goldbert NS, Robinson JR, Roenick HH. Plasmapharesis in bullous pemphigoid. *Arch Dermatol* 1985;121:1484–5

37. Cropley T, Ahmed AR. Bullous Diseases. In Newcomer VD, Young EM, eds. *Geriatric Dermatology*. New York: Igaku-Shoin Med. Publishers, 1989:151–69

38. Axt M, Wever S, Baier G, *et al*. Cicatricial pemphigoid – therapeutic problem. Review. (German) *Hautarzt* 1995;46:620–7

39. Ahmed RR, Kurgis BS, Rogers RS. Cicatricial pemphigoid (clinical review). *J Am Acad Dermatol* 1991;24:987–1001

40. Mutasim DF, Pelc NJ, Anhalt GJ. Cicatricial pemphigoid: bullous diseases. *Dermatol Clin* 1993;11:499–510

41. Kurzhals G, Maciejewski W, Agathos M, *et al*. Localized cicatricial bullous pemphigoid of the Brunsting–Perry type. (German) *Hautarzt* 1993;44:110–13

42. Flotte TJ. Pathology of bullous pemphigoid. *Clin Dermatol* 1987;5:71–80

43. Medved A, Maxwell I. Intermittent cyclophosphamide in pemphigus vulgaris and bullous pemphigoid. *Can Med Assoc J* 1974;111:245–50

44. Gammon WR, Briggaman RA. Epidermolysis bullosa acquisita and bullous systemic lupus erythematosus: diseases of autoimmunity to type VII collagen: bullous diseases. *Dermatol Clin* 1993;11:535–47

45. Muller SA, Sams WM, Dobson RL. Amyloidosis masquerading as epidermolysis bullosa acquisita. *Arch Dermatol* 1969;99:739–47

46. Metz G, Metz J, Frank H. Epidermolysis bullosa aquissita bei morbus crohn. *Hautarzt* 1975;26:321–6

47. Roenigk HH, Roenigk HR, Ryan JC, Bergfeld WR. Epidermolysis bullosa acquisita. *Arch Dermatol* 1971;103:1–10

48. Woodley DT, Gammon WR, Briggaman RA. Epidermolysis bullosa acquisita: autoimmunity to type VII collagen. In Fitzpatrick TB, Eisen AZ, Wolff K, *et al*., eds. *Dermatology in General Medicine*, 5th edn. New York: McGraw-Hill, 1993:702–8

49. Pehr K, Forsey RR. Why don't we use Vit E in dermatology? *Can Med Assoc J* 1993;149: 1247–53

50. Gordon KB, Chan LS, Woodley DT. Treatment of refractory epidermolysis bullosa acquisita with extracorporeal photochemotherapy. *Br J Dermatol* 1997;136:415–20

51. Smith EP, Zone, JJ. Dermatitis herpetiformis and linear IgA bullous dermatosis: bullous diseases. *Dermatol Clin* 1993;11:511–526

52. Katz SI, Hall RP, Lawlwey TJ, *et al*. Dermatitis herpetiformis: the skin and the gut. *Ann Intern Med* 1980;98:857

53. Katz SI. Dermatitis herpetiformis. In Fitzpatrick TB, Eisen AZ, Wolff K, *et al*., eds. *Dermatology in General Medicine*, 5th edn. New York: McGraw-Hill, 1993:636–41

54. Mutasim DF, Pelc NJ, Supapannachrt N. Established methods in the investigation of bullous diseases: bullous diseases. *Dermatol Clin* 1993;11:399–418

55. Tan CC, Sale JE, Brammer C, *et al*. Dapsone: modes of action, toxicity and possible strategies for increasing patient tolerance. Review. *Br J Dermatol* 1993;139:507–13

56. Zemtsov A, Neldner KH. Successful treatment of dermatitis herpetiformis with tetracycline and nicotinamide in a patient unable to tolerate dapsone. *J Am Acad Dermatol* 1993;28: 505–6

57. Garioch JJ, Lewis HM, Sargent SA, *et al*. 25 years experience on a gluten free diet in the treatment of dermatitis herpetiformis. *Br J Dermatol* 1994;131:541–5

58. Rackett SC, Rothe MJ, Grant-Kels JM, *et al*. Diet and dermatology: the role of dietary manipulation in the prevention and treatment of cutaneous disorders. *J Am Acad Dermatol* 1993;29:447–61

59. Harber LC, Bickers DR. The porphyrias. In *Photosensitivity Diseases: Principles of Diagnosis and Treatment*, 2nd edn. Philadelphia: BC Decker, 1989:241–87

60. De Verneuil H, Aitken G, Nordmann Y. Familial and sporadic porphyria cutanea tarda: two different diseases. *Hum Genet* 1974;44: 145–51

61. Elder GH. Porphyria cutanea tarda: a multifactorial disease. In Champion RH, Pye RJ, eds. *Recent Advances in Dermatology*, Vol 8. Edinburgh: Churchill Livingstone, 1990:55–69

62. Grossman ME, Poh-Fitzpatrick MB. Porphyria cutanea tarda: diagnosis, management, and differentiation from other hepatic porphyrias. *Dermatol Clin* 1986;4:297–309

63. Grossman ME, Bickers DR, Poh-Fitzpatrick MB, *et al*. Porphyria cutanea tarda: clinical features and laboratory findings in 40 patients. *Am J Med* 1979;67:277–86

64. Lamkin BC, Bickers DR. Porphyria cutanea tarda: a metabolic human blistering disease. *Dermatol Clin* 1983;1:249–62

65. Cormane RH, Szabo E, Hoo TT. Histopathology of the skin in acquired and hereditary

porphyria cutanea tarda. *Br J Dermatol* 1971;85:531–9

66. Gilchrest B, Rowe JW, Mihm MC. Bullous dermatosis of hemodialysis. *Ann Intern Med* 1975;83:480–3

67. Saltzer EI, Redeker AG, Wilson JW. Porphyria cutanea tarda: remission following chloroquine administration without adverse effects. *Arch Dermatol* 1968;98:496–8

68. Richards SS, Hall S, Yokel B, *et al*. A bullous eruption in an elderly woman: vancomycin associated linear IgA dermatosis (LAD). *Arch Dermatol* 1995;131:1447–8, 1450–1

69. Chaffins ML, Collison D, Fivenson DP. Treatment of pemphigus and linear IgA dermatosis with nicotinamide and tetracycline: a review of 13 cases. *J Am Acad Dermatol* 1993;28:998–9

70. Taniguchi Y, Wada Y, Takahashi M, *et al*. Multiple bullae and paresis after drug-induced coma. *Acta Derm Venereol* 1991;71:536–8

71. Torne R, Soyer HP, Leb G, *et al*. Skin lesions in carbon monoxide intoxication. *Dermatologica* 1991;183:212–15

72. Holden CE. Cutaneous bullae in coma due to poisoning. An association with deep seated ischemic lesions of the muscle. *Anaesthesia* 1977;32:554–5

73. Wenzel FG, Horn D. Non-neoplastic disorders of the eccrine glands. *J Am Acad Dermatol* 1998;38:1–17

74. Mehregan DR, Daoud M, Rogers RS. Coma blisters in a patient with diabetic ketoacidosis. *J Am Acad Dermatol* 1992;27:269–70

75. Arndt KA, Mihm MC Jr, Parrish JA. Bullae: a cutaneous sign of a variety of neurologic diseases. *J Invest Dermatol* 1973;60:312–20

76. Leavell UW Jr, Coyer JR, Taylor RJ. Dermographism and erythematous lines in glutethimide overdose. *Arch Dermatol* 1972; 106:724–5

77. Sanchez Yus E, Requena L, Simon P, *et al*. Histopathology of cutaneous changes in drug-induced coma. Review. *Am J Dermatopathol* 1993;15:208–16

78. Honigsmann H, Trautinger F, Wolff K. Subcorneal pustular dermatosis (Sneddon–Wilkinson Disease). In Fitzpatrick TB, Eisen AZ, Wolff K, *et al.*, eds. *Dermatology in General Medicine*, 5th edn. New York: McGraw-Hill, 1999:719–22

79. Grover RW. Transient acantholytic dermatosis. *Arch Dermatol* 1970;101:426–34

80. Ackerman AB. Focal acantholytic dyskeratosis. *Arch Dermatol* 1972;106:702–6

81. Heenan PJ, Quirk CJ. Transient acantholytic dermatosis (Grover's disease). In Fitzpatrick TB, Eisen AZ, Wolff K, *et al.*, eds. *Dermatology in General Medicine*, 5th edn. New York: McGraw-Hill, 1999:620–3

Adverse drug reactions on the skin 9

J. Z. Litt

INTRODUCTION

Adverse drug reactions are the 'diseases of medical progress', the inevitable price we pay for the benefits of modern drug therapy. The side-effects of drugs cannot be avoided. In 42 BCE Publilius Syrus averred: 'There are some remedies worse than the disease'!

It is an inescapable truth that more and more people – primarily the older population – are taking more and more over-the-counter and prescription medications. New drugs for all types of disorders – high blood pressure, gastric ulcers, diabetes, migraine, high cholesterol, etc. – are appearing in the medical market place on an almost daily basis. Unfortunately, more and more drug reactions, primarily on the skin, hair, nails and mucous membranes, have been increasing from many of these medications. Who, for example, does not take aspirin, acetaminophen or ibuprofen? Who is not treated with an antibiotic when suffering from some bacterial or viral infection? How many elderly patients are being treated with a beta-blocker, an ACE-inhibitor, an antidepressant or a non-steroidal anti-inflammatory drug (NSAID)? There is not a medication in the market place that cannot give rise to some form of drug reaction in certain unfortunate sensitive individuals. According to the World Health Organization definition, 'Adverse drug reactions are any noxious, unintended, and undesired effects of a drug which occur at doses used in humans for prophylaxis, diagnosis, or therapy'. Adverse reactions which result from immunologic responses to drugs or their metabolites are important causes of morbidity and mortality. Adverse reactions to prescription drugs are the fourth greatest cause of death in the USA (after heart disease, cancer, and stroke); it is estimated that more than 100 000 Americans die every year as a result of such reactions.

A hundred years ago there were not that many drugs to cause adverse cutaneous reactions and there was only one drug 'eruption' book published in the 19th century. Since 1950, systemic drug therapy has increased enormously, and a whole new series of morphologically variable adverse effects has been observed.

SKIN REACTIONS

Skin reactions are the most frequent manifestation of drug sensitivity. A variety of cutaneous adverse reactions, from mild, maculopapular eruptions to severe, life-threatening conditions, such as Stevens–Johnson syndrome, toxic epidermal necrolysis, exfoliative dermatitis, anaphylaxis, serum-sickness, hypersensitivity reactions and others, may be caused by drugs. Systemically administered drugs can produce various kinds of skin reaction. The same drug may give rise to several types of reaction pattern, and many different drugs may induce morphologically similar skin reactions.

The incidence of adverse reactions specific to a drug will generally be related to the frequency of the drug prescribed and the total amount of it used. The current estimate is that 2 to 3% of the general population and 15 to 30% of hospitalized patients develop severe adverse reactions to drugs. This disparity arises because hospitalized patients are usually older and are given more and different classes of medication.

Drug eruptions, those adverse side-effects on the skin, hair, nails and mucous membranes, can take on the appearance typical of almost any dermatologic entity. They used to say that syphilis was the 'great mimicker'. Now it is the drug eruption that is the great mimicker. Undesirable drug reactions – the incidence of which is increased in AIDS patients – may appear within minutes, for example urticaria or anaphylactic shock after penicillin; or they may take several days, weeks, or months to appear, for example purpura or exfoliative dermatitis or lichenoid eruptions after penicillamine or gold.

An adverse cutaneous reaction to a drug may be suspected when the use of a medication – usually the last new drug the patient has taken – is closely followed by one of the classic morphologic patterns associated with drug eruptions (exanthems, urticaria, FXE, photosensitivity, etc.) or when a pre-existing skin disease worsens in a patient taking a drug that is known to cause such exacerbations, such as lithium and acne or lithium and psoriasis; oral contraceptives and acne; phenytoin and gingival hyperplasia, and others. If a sudden, pruritic, symmetrical rash appears, a drug eruption must be first on the differential diagnosis list.

The following 29 reaction patterns, listed in alphabetical order, are some of the most common adverse side-effects from medications.

Acanthosis nigricans

Acanthosis nigricans (AN) is a process characterized by a soft, velvety, brown or grayish-black thickening of the skin that is symmetrically distributed over the axillae, neck, inguinal areas and other body folds (see Chapter 3, Figure 32). While most cases of AN are seen in obese and prepubertal children, it can occur as a marker for various endocrinopathies as well as in female patients with elevated testosterone levels, irregular menses and hirsutism. It is frequently a concomitant of an underlying malignant condition, principally an adenocarcinoma of the intestinal tract.

Responsible drugs include cortisone, lithium, and oral contraceptives.

Acneform lesions

Acneform eruptions are inflammatory follicular reactions that resemble acne vulgaris and that are manifested clinically as papules or pustules. They are monomorphic reactions, have a monomorphic appearance, and are found primarily on the upper parts of the body. Unlike acne vulgaris, there are rarely comedones present. A drug-induced acneform eruption may be suspected if:

(1) The onset is sudden;
(2) There is a worsening of existing acne lesions;
(3) The extent is considerable from the outset;
(4) The appearance is monomorphic;
(5) The localization is unusual for acne as, for example, when the distal extremities are involved;
(6) The patient's age is unusual for regular acne; and
(7) There is exposure to a potentially responsible drug.

The most common drugs responsible for acneform eruptions are: adrenocorticotropic hormone (ACTH), androgenic hormones, anti-convulsants (hydantoin derivatives, phenobarbital, trimethadione), corticosteroids, danazol, disulfiram, halides (bromides, chlorides, iodides), lithium, oral contraceptives, tuberculostatics (ethionamide, isoniazid, rifampin) and vitamins B_2, B_6 and B_{12}.

Acute generalized exanthematous pustulosis

Arising on the face or intertriginous areas, acute generalized exanthematous pustulosis (AGEP) is characterized by a rapidly evolving, widespread, scarlatiniform eruption covered with hundreds of small superficial pustules. Often accompanied by a high fever, AGEP is most frequently associated with penicillin and macrolide antibiotics, and usually occurs within 24 hours of exposure to the drug.

Alopecia

Many drugs have been reported to cause hair loss. Commonly appearing as a diffuse alopecia, it affects women more frequently than men and is limited in most instances to the scalp. Axillary and pubic hairs are rarely affected except with anticoagulants.

The hair loss from cytostatic agents, which is dose-dependent and begins about two weeks after the onset of therapy, is a result of the interruption of the anagen (growing) cycle of hair. With other drugs the hair loss does not begin until 2 to 5 months after the medication has been started. With cholesterol-lowering drugs, diffuse alopecia is a result of interference with normal keratinization. The scalp is normal and drug-induced alopecia is almost always reversible within one to three months after the therapy has been discontinued. The regrown hair is frequently depigmented and occasionally more curly.

The most frequent offenders are cytostatic agents and anticoagulants, but hair loss can occur with a variety of common drugs, including hormones, anticonvulsants, amantadine, amiodarone, captopril, cholesterol-lowering drugs, cimetidine, colchicine, etretinate, isotretinoin, ketoconazole, heavy metals, lithium, penicillamine, valproic acid and propranolol.

Angioedema

Angioedema is the term applied to a variant of urticaria in which the subcutaneous tissues, rather than the dermis, are mainly involved. Also known as Quincke's edema, giant urticaria and angioneurotic edema, this acute, evanescent, skin-colored, circumscribed edema usually affects the most distensible tissues: the lips, eyelids, earlobes and genitalia. It can also affect the mucous membranes of the tongue, mouth and larynx. Symptoms of angioedema, frequently unilateral, asymmetrical and non-pruritic, generally last for an hour or two but can persist for 2 to 5 days.

The etiological factors associated with angioedema are as varied as that of urticaria (see below).

Aphthous stomatitis

Aphthous stomatitis – also known as canker sores – is a common disease of the oral mucous membranes. Arising as tiny, discrete or grouped, papules or vesicles, these painful lesions develop into small (2–5 mm in diameter), round, shallow ulcerations having a grayish, yellow base surrounded by a thin red border. Located predominantly over the labial and buccal mucosae, these aphthae heal without scarring in 10 to 14 days. Recurrences are common.

The most common offenders are aspirin, captopril, diflunisal, gold, ibuprofen, naproxen, paroxetine, sulfamethoxale, and terbinafine.

Black hairy tongue

Black hairy tongue (BHT) (lingua villosa nigra) presents as benign hyperplasia of the filiform papillae of the anterior two-thirds of the tongue. These papillary elongations, usually associated with black, brown, or yellow pigmentation attributed to the overgrowth of pigment-producing bacteria, may be as long as 2 cm. Occurring only in adults, BHT has been associated with the administration of oral antibiotics, poor dental hygiene and excessive smoking.

Bullous eruptions

Bullous and vesicular drug eruptions are diseases in which blisters and vesicles occur as a complication of the administration of drugs. Blisters are a well-known manifestation of cutaneous reactions to drugs. In many types of drug reaction bullae and vesicles may be found in addition to other manifestations. Bullae are usually noted in erythema multiforme, Stevens–Johnson syndrome, toxic epidermal necrolysis, fixed eruptions when very intense, urticaria, vasculitis, porphyria cutanea tarda and phototoxic reactions (from furosemide and nalidixic acid). Tense, thick-walled bullae can be seen in bromoderma and iododerma as well as in barbiturate overdosage.

Common drugs that cause bullous eruptions and bullous pemphigoid (see Chapter 8, Figure 6) are: nadalol, penicillamine, piroxi-cam, psoralens, rifampin, clonidine, furo-semide, diclofenac, mefenamic acid, bleomycin and others.

Erythema multiforme and Stevens–Johnson syndrome

Erythema multiforme is a relatively common, acute, self-limited, inflammatory reaction pat-tern that is often associated with a preceding herpes simplex or mycoplasma infection. Other causes are associated with connective tissue disease, physical agents, X-ray therapy, pregnancy and internal malignancies, to mention a few. In 50% of the cases no cause can be found. In a recent prospective study of erythema multiforme, only 10% were drug related. The eruption rapidly occurs over a period of 12 to 24 hours. In about half the cases there are prodromal symptoms of an upper respiratory infection accompanied by fever, malaise and varying degrees of muscu-lar and joint pains. Clinically, bluish-red, well-demarcated, macular, papular, or urticarial lesions, as well as the classical 'iris' or 'target lesions', sometimes with central vesicles, bul-lae, or purpura, are distributed preferentially over the distal extremities, especially over the dorsa of the hands and extensor aspects of the forearms. Lesions tend to spread peripherally and may involve the palms and trunk as well as the mucous membranes of the mouth and genitalia. Central healing and overlapping lesions often lead to arciform, annular and gyrate patterns. Lesions appear over the course of a week or ten days and resolve over the next two weeks.

The Stevens–Johnson syndrome, a severe and occasionally fatal variety of erythema multiforme, has an abrupt onset and is accompanied by any or all of the following: fever, myalgia, malaise, headache, arthralgia and ocular involvement, with occasional bullae and erosions covering less than 10% of the body surface. Painful stomatitis is an early and conspicuous symptom. Hemorrhagic bullae may appear over the lips, mouth and genital mucous membranes. Patients are often acutely ill with high fever. The course from eruption to healing of the lesions may extend up to six weeks.

The following drugs have been most often associated with erythema multiforme and Stevens–Johnson syndrome: allopurinol, anti-convulsants (phenytoin), barbiturates, carba-mazepine, estrogens/progestins, gold, NSAIDs, penicillamine, sulfonamides, tetracycline and tolbutamide.

Erythema nodosum

Erythema nodosum is a cutaneous reaction pattern characterized by erythematous, ten-der or painful subcutaneous nodules com-monly distributed over the anterior aspect of the lower legs, and occasionally elsewhere. More common in young women, erythema nodosum is often associated with increased estrogen levels such as occur during preg-nancy and with the ingestion of oral contra-ceptives. It is also an occasional manifestation of streptococcal infection, sarcoidosis, sec-ondary syphilis, tuberculosis, certain deep fun-gal infections, Hodgkin's disease, leukemia, ulcerative colitis and radiation therapy and is often preceded by fever, fatigue, arthralgia, vomiting and diarrhea. The incidence of ery-thema nodosum due to drugs is low and it is impossible to distinguish clinically between erythema nodosum due to drugs and that caused by other factors.

Some of the drugs that are known to cause erythema nodosum are: antibiotics, estrogens, amiodarone, gold, NSAIDs, oral contracep-tives, sulfonamides and opiates.

Exanthems

Exanthems, commonly resembling viral rashes, represent the most common type of cutaneous drug eruption. Described as macu-lopapular or morbilliform eruptions, these flat, barely raised, erythematous patches, from one to several millimeters in diameter, are usually bilateral and symmetrical. They commonly begin on the head and neck or upper torso and progress downward to the limbs. They may present or develop into confluent areas and may be accompanied by pruritus and a mild fever. The exanthems caused by drugs can be classified as either morbilliform eruptions (fingernail-sized erythematous patches) or scarlatiniform eruptions, which are punctate, pinpoint, or pinhead-sized lesions in erythematous areas that have a tendency to coalesce. Circumoral pallor and the subsequent appearance of scaling may also be noted.

Maculopapular drug eruptions usually fade with desquamation and, occasionally, post-inflammatory hyperpigmentation, in about two weeks. They invariably recur on rechal-lenge. Exanthems often have a sudden onset during the first two weeks of administration, except for those caused by semi-synthetic penicillins, which frequently develop after the first two weeks following the initial dose.

The drugs most commonly associated with exanthems are: amoxicillin, ampicillin, bleomycin, captopril, carbamazepine, chlor-promazine, cotrimoxazole, gold, nalidixic acid, naproxen, phenytoin, penicillamine and piroxicam.

Exfoliative dermatitis

Exfoliative dermatitis is a rare but serious reaction pattern that is characterized by ery-thema, pruritus and scaling over the entire body (erythroderma; see Chapter 3, Figure 31). Drug-induced exfoliative dermatitis usually begins a few weeks or longer following the administration of a culpable drug. Beginning as erythematous, edematous patches, often on the face, it spreads to involve the entire integument. The skin becomes swollen and scarlet and may ooze a straw-colored fluid; this is followed in a few days by desquama-tion. High fever, severe malaise and chills,

along with enlargement of the lymph nodes, often coexist with the cutaneous changes.

One of the most dangerous of all reac-tion patterns, exfoliative dermatitis can be accompanied by any or all of the following: hypothermia, fluid and electrolyte loss, cardiac failure and gastrointestinal hemor-rhage. Death may supervene if the drug is continued after the onset of the eruption. Secondary infection often complicates the course of the disease. Once the active der-matitis has receded, hyperpigmentation as well as loss of hair and nails may ensue.

The following drugs, among others, can bring about exfoliative dermatitis: barbitu-rates, captopril, carbamazepine, cimetidine, furosemide, gold, isoniazid, lithium, nitro-furantoin, NSAIDs, penicillamine, phenytoin, pyrazolones, quinidine, streptomycin, sulfon-amides and thiazides.

Fixed eruptions

A fixed eruption is an unusual hypersensitivity reaction characterized by one or more well-demarcated erythematous plaques that recur at the same cutaneous (or mucosal) site or sites each time exposure to the offending agent occurs. The size of the lesions varies from a few millimeters to as much as twenty centimeters in diameter. Almost any drug that is ingested, injected, inhaled, or inserted into the body can trigger this skin reaction. The eruption typically begins as a sharply marginated, solitary edematous papule or plaque – occasionally surmounted by a large bulla – which usually develops 30 minutes to 8 hours following the administration of a drug. If the offending agent is not promptly eliminated, the inflammation intensifies, pro-ducing a dusky red, violaceous or brown patch that may crust, desquamate, or blister within 7 to 10 days. The lesions are rarely pruritic. Favored sites are the hands, feet, face and genitalia – especially the glans penis.

The reason for the specific localization of the skin lesions in a fixed drug eruption is unknown. The offending drug cannot be detected at the skin site. Certain drugs cause a fixed eruption at specific sites, for example tetracycline and ampicillin often elicit a fixed eruption on the penis, whereas aspirin usually causes skin lesions on the face, limbs and trunk.

Common causes of fixed eruptions are: ampicillin, aspirin, barbiturates, dapsone, metronidazole, NSAIDs, oral contraceptives, phenolphthalein, phenytoin, quinine, sulfonamides and tetracyclines.

Gingival hyperplasia

Gingival hyperplasia, a common, undesirable, non-allergic drug reaction, begins as a diffuse swelling of the interdental papillae. Particularly prevalent with phenytoin therapy, gingival hyperplasia begins about three months after the onset of therapy and occurs in 30 to 70% of patients receiving it. The severity of the reaction is dose-dependent and children and young adults are more frequently affected. The most severe cases are noted in young women. In many cases gingival hyperplasia is accompanied by painful and bleeding gums. There is often superimposed secondary bacterial gingivitis. This can be so extensive that the teeth of the maxilla and mandible are completely overgrown.

While it is characteristically a side-effect of hydantoin derivatives, it may occur during the administration of phenobarbital, nifedipine, diltiazem and other medications.

Lichenoid (lichen planus-like) eruptions

Lichenoid eruptions are so called because of their resemblance to lichen planus, a papulosquamous disorder that characteristically presents as multiple, discrete, violaceous, flat-topped papules, often polygonal in shape, which are extremely pruritic. Not infrequently, lichenoid lesions appear weeks or months following exposure to the responsible drug. As a rule, the symptoms begin to recede a few weeks following the discontinuation of the drug.

Common drug causes of lichenoid eruptions are: antimalarials, beta-blockers, chlorpropamide, furosemide, gold, methyldopa, phenothiazines, quinidine, thiazides and tolazamide.

Lupus erythematosus

A reaction clinically and pathologically resembling idiopathic systemic lupus erythematosus (SLE) has been reported in association with a large variety of drugs. There is some evidence that drug-induced SLE, invariably accompanied by a positive ANA reaction with 90% having antihistone antibodies, may have a genetically determined basis. These symptoms of SLE, a relatively benign form of lupus, recede within days or weeks following the discontinuation of the responsible drug. Skin lesions occur in about 20% of cases. Drugs cause fewer than 8% of all cases of systemic lupus erythematosus.

The following drugs have been commonly associated with inducing, aggravating or unmasking SLE: beta-blockers, carbamazepine, chlorpromazine, estrogens, griseofulvin, hydralazine, isoniazid (INH), lithium, methyldopa, minoxidil, oral contraceptives, penicillamine, phenytoin (diphenylhydantoin), procainamide, propylthiouracil, quinidine and testosterone.

Onycholysis

Onycholysis, the painless separation of the nail plate from the nail bed, is one of the most common nail disorders (see Chapter 5). The unattached portion, which is white and opaque, usually begins at the free margin and proceeds proximally, causing part or most of the nail plate to become separated. The attached, healthy portion of the nail, by contrast, is pink and translucent.

Responsible drugs include allopurinol, captopril, doxycycline, ibuprofen, oral contraceptives and tetracycline.

Pemphigus vulgaris

Pemphigus vulgaris (PV) is a rare, serious, acute or chronic, blistering disease involving the skin and mucous membranes (see

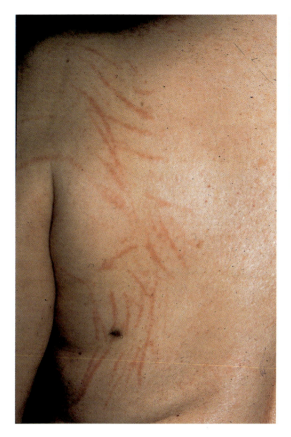

Figure 1   Scratch excoriation secondary to pruritus

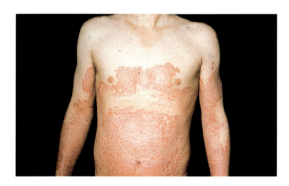

Figure 2   Psoriasis exacerbation secondary to a drug reaction

Chapter 8, Figures 1 and 2). Characterized by thin-walled, easily-ruptured, flaccid bullae that are seen to arise on normal or erythematous skin and over mucous membranes, the lesions of PV appear initially in the mouth (in about 60% of cases) and then spread, after

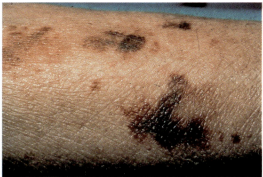

Figure 3   Drug-induced purpura

weeks or months, to involve the axillae and groin, the scalp, face and neck. The lesions may become generalized. Because of their fragile roofs the bullae rupture leaving painful erosions, and crusts may develop principally over the scalp.

Responsible drugs include acetaminophen, amoxicillin, aspirin, phenobarbital and propranolol.

Photosensitivity

A photosensitive reaction is a chemically-induced change in the skin that makes an individual unusually sensitive to light. On absorbing light of a specific wavelength, an oral, injected or topical drug may be chemically altered to produce a reaction ranging from macules and papules, vesicles and bullae, edema, urticaria, or an acute eczematous reaction. Any eruption that is prominent on the face, the dorsa of the hands, the 'V' of the neck and the presternal area should suggest an adverse reaction to light. The distribution is the key to the diagnosis. Initially the eruption, which consists of erythema, edema, blisters, weeping and desquamation, involves the forehead, rims of the ears, the nose, the malar eminences and cheeks, the sides and back of the neck, the extensor surfaces of the forearms and the dorsa of the hands. These reactions commonly spare the shaded areas: those under the chin, under the nose, behind the ears and inside the fold of the upper eyelids.

There is usually a sharp cut-off at the site of jewelry and at clothing margins. All light-exposed areas need not be affected equally.

There are two main types of photosensitive reaction: the phototoxic and the photoallergic reaction. Phototoxic reactions, the most common type of drug-induced photosensitivity, resemble an exaggerated sunburn and occur within 5 to 20 hours after the skin has been exposed to a photosensitizing substance and light of the proper wavelength and intensity. It is not a form of allergy – prior sensitization is not required – and, theoretically, could occur in anyone given enough drug and light. Phototoxic reactions are dose-dependent both for drug and sunlight. Patients with phototoxicity reactions are commonly sensitive to ultraviolet A (UVA radiation), the so-called 'tanning rays' at 320–400 nm. Phototoxic reactions may cause onycholysis, as the nailbed is particularly susceptible because of its lack of melanin protection.

Patients with a true photoallergy (the interaction of drug, light and the immune system), a less common form of drug-induced photosensitivity, are often sensitive to UVB radiation, the so-called 'burning rays' at 290–320 nm. Photoallergic reactions, unlike phototoxic responses, represent an immunologic change and require a latent period of from 24 to 48 hours, during which sensitization occurs. They are not dose-related. If the photosensitizer acts internally, it is a photo-drug reaction; if it acts externally, it is photo-contact dermatitis.

Drugs that are likely to cause phototoxic reactions are: amiodarone, nalidixic acid, various NSAIDs, phenothiazines (especially chlorpromazine) and tetracyclines (particularly demeclocycline). Photoallergic reactions may occur as a result of exposure to systemically-administered drugs such as griseofulvin, NSAIDs, phenothiazines, quinidine, sulfonamides, sulfonylureas and thiazide diuretics as well as to external agents such as para-aminobenzoic acid (found in sunscreens), bithionol (used in soaps and cosmetics), para-phenylenediamine and others.

Pigmentation

Drug-induced pigmentation on the skin, hair, nails and mucous membranes is a result of either melanin synthesis, increased lipofuscin synthesis, or post-inflammatory pigmentation. Color changes, which can be localized or widespread, can also result from deposition of bile pigments (jaundice), exogenous metal compounds, and direct deposition of compounds such as carotene or quinacrine. Post-inflammatory pigmentation can follow a variety of drug-induced inflammatory cutaneous reactions; fixed eruptions are known to leave a residual pigmentation that can persist for months.

The following is a partial list of those drugs that can cause various pigmentary changes: anticonvulsants, antimalarials, cytostatics, hormones, metals, tetracyclines, phenothiazine tranquilizers, psoralens, amiodarone, etc.

Pityriasis rosea-like eruptions

Pityriasis rosea, commonly mistaken for ringworm, is a unique disorder that usually begins as a single, large, round or oval pinkish patch known as the 'mother' or 'herald' patch. The most common sites for this solitary lesion are the chest, the back, or the abdomen. This is followed in about two weeks by a blossoming of small, flat, round or oval, scaly patches of similar color, each with a central collarette scale, usually distributed in a Christmas tree-like pattern over the trunk and, to a lesser degree, the extremities. This eruption seldom itches and usually limits itself to areas from the neck to the knees. In drug-induced pityriasis rosea, the 'herald patch' is usually absent, and the eruption will often not follow the classic pattern.

While the etiology of idiopathic pityriasis rosea is unknown, we do know that various medications have been reported to give rise to this benign disorder. These are: barbiturates, beta-blockers, bismuth, captopril, clonidine, gold, griseofulvin, isotretinoin, labetalol, meprobamate, metronidazole, penicillin and tripelennamine.

Pruritus

Generalized itching, without any visible signs of irritation, is one of the least common adverse reactions to drugs. More frequently than not, drug-induced itching – moderate or severe – is fairly generalized (Figure 1). For most drugs it is not known how they elicit pruritus; some drugs can cause itching directly or indirectly through cholestasis. Pruritus may develop by different pathogenetic mechanisms: allergic, pseudoallergic (histamine release), neurogenic, by vasodilatation, cholestatic effect and others.

A partial list of those drugs that can cause pruritus is: aspirin, NSAIDs, penicillins, sulfonamides, chloroquine, ACE inhibitors, amiodarone, nicotinic acid derivatives, lithium, bleomycin, tamoxifen, interferons, gold, penicillamine, methoxsalen, isotretinoin, etc.

Psoriasis

Many drugs, as a result of their pharmacological action, have been implicated in the precipitation or exacerbation of psoriasis or psoriasiform eruptions. Psoriasis is a common, chronic, papulosquamous disorder of unknown etiology with characteristic histopathological features and many biochemical, physiological and immunological abnormalities (Figure 2).

Drugs that can precipitate psoriasis are, among others, beta-blockers and lithium. Drugs that are reported to aggravate psoriasis are antimalarials, beta-blockers, lithium, NSAIDs, quinidine and photosensitizing drugs. The effect and extent of these drug-induced psoriatic eruptions are dose dependent.

Purpura

Purpura, a result of hemorrhage into the skin, can be divided into thrombocytopenic purpura and non-thrombocytopenic purpura (vascular purpura) (Figure 3). Both thrombocytopenic and vascular purpura may be due to drugs, and most of the drugs producing purpura may do so by giving rise to vascular damage and thrombocytopenia. In both types of purpura, allergic or toxic (non-allergic) mechanisms may be involved. Some drugs combine with platelets to form an antigen, stimulating formation of antibody to the platelet–drug combination. Thus the drug appears to act as a hapten; subsequent antigen–antibody reaction causes platelet destruction leading to thrombocytopenia. Purpuric lesions are usually more marked over the lower portions of the body, notably the legs and dorsal aspects of the feet in ambulatory patients. Other drug-induced cutaneous reactions – erythema multiforme, erythema nodosum, fixed eruption, necrotizing vasculitis and others – can have a prominent purpuric component.

A whole host of drugs can give rise to purpura, the most common being: NSAIDs, thiazide diuretics, phenothiazines, cytostatics, gold, penicillamine, hydantoins, thiouracils and sulfonamides.

Raynaud's phenomenon

Raynaud's phenomenon is the paroxysmal, cold-induced constriction of small arteries and arterioles of the fingers and, less often, the toes. Occurring more frequently in women, Raynaud's phenomenon is characterized by blanching, pallor and cyanosis. In severe cases secondary changes may occur: thinning and ridging of the nails, telangiectases of the nail folds, and, in the later stages, sclerosis and atrophy of the digits.

Offending drugs include: clonidine, beta-blockers, bleomycin, cyclosporine, minocycline, spironolactone, and vincristine.

Toxic epidermal necrolysis

Also known as Lyell's syndrome and the scalded skin syndrome, toxic epidermal necrolysis (TEN) is a rare, serious, acute exfoliative, bullous eruption of the skin and mucous membranes that usually develops as a reaction to diverse drugs. TEN can also be a result of a bacterial or viral infection and can develop after radiation therapy or vaccinations. In the drug-induced form of TEN, a morbilliform eruption accompanied by large, red, tender areas of the skin will develop shortly after the drug has been administered. This progresses rapidly to blistering, and a widespread exfoliation of the epidermis develops dramatically over a very short period, accompanied by high fever. The hairy parts of the body are usually spared. The mucous membranes and eyes are often involved. The clinical picture resembles an extensive second-degree burn and the patient is acutely ill. Fatigue, vomiting, diarrhea and angina are prodromal symptoms. In a few hours the condition becomes grave. Toxic epidermal necrolysis is a medical emergency, and unless the offending agent is discontinued immediately, the outcome may be fatal in the course of a few days.

Drugs that are the most common cause of TEN are: allopurinol, ampicillin, amoxicillin, carbamazepine, NSAIDs, phenobarbital, pentamidine, phenytoin (diphenylhydantoin), pyrazolones and sulfonamides.

Urticaria

Urticaria induced by drugs is, after exanthems, the second most common type of drug reaction. Urticaria, or hives, is a vascular reaction of the skin characterized by pruritic, erythematous wheals. These wheals or welts, caused by localized edema, can vary in size from one millimeter in diameter to large palm-sized swellings, favor the covered areas (trunk, buttocks, chest), and are, more often than not, generalized. Urticaria usually develops within 36 hours following the administration of the responsible drug. Individual lesions rarely persist for more than 24 hours. Urticaria may be the only symptom of drug sensitivity, or it may be a concomitant or be followed by the manifestations of serum sickness. Urticaria may be accompanied by angioedema of the lips or eyelids. It may, on rare occasions, progress to anaphylactoid reactions or to anaphylaxis.

The following are the most common causes of drug-induced urticaria: antibiotics, notably penicillin (more commonly following parenteral administration than by ingestion), barbiturates, captopril, levamisole, NSAIDs, quinine, rifampin, sulfonamides, thiopental and vancomycin.

Vasculitis

Drug-induced cutaneous necrotizing vasculitis, a clinicopathologic process characterized by inflammation and necrosis of blood vessels, often presents with a variety of small, palpable purpuric lesions most frequently distributed over the lower extremities: urticaria-like lesions, small ulcerations and occasional hemorrhagic vesicles and pustules. The basic process involves an immunologically mediated response to antigens that results in damage to the vessel walls. Beginning as small macules and papules, they ultimately result in purpuric lesions and, in more severe cases, into hemorrhagic blisters and frank ulcerations. A polymorphonuclear infiltrate and fibrinoid changes in the small dermal vessels characterize the vasculitic reaction.

Drugs that are commonly associated with vasculitis are: ACE-inhibitors, amiodarone, ampicillin, cimetidine, coumadin, furosemide, hydantoins, hydralazine, NSAIDs, pyrazolones, quinidine, sulfonamides, thiazides and thiouracils.

Xerostomia

Xerostomia is a dryness of the oral cavity that makes speaking, chewing and swallowing difficult. Resulting from a partial or complete absence of saliva production, xerostomia can be caused by a variety of medications.

Leg ulcers: diagnostic approach and management

10

A. I. Rojas, Y. M. Bello and T. J. Phillips

INTRODUCTION

Leg ulcers are a common problem and tend to affect the elderly population, although they can occur at any age. As the population ages the prevalence of leg ulcers is increasing[1–3]. Limited epidemiological data are available from the United States. Data from the 1990 surveys by the National Center for Health Statistics, Center of Disease Control, showed that venous ulceration occurred in 300 000 patients[4]. More accurate epidemiological data about leg ulcers come from European countries, where leg ulcers may affect between 0.11 and 1% of the population[5,6]. Leg ulcers are frequently a chronic condition in which, as observed by Nelzen and colleagues, as many as 50% of patients had their first ulcer before the age of 65, with the highest prevalence of open venous ulcers observed in patients older than 70[1].

Venous insufficiency is the most common cause of leg ulcers, accounting for 54–81% of them[1–3,7,8], followed by mixed venous and arterial disease (14–26%)[1,3,8]. Arterial disease accounts for 5–18% of ulcers and is frequently associated with diabetic neuropathy[8]. Diabetic neuropathic ulcers alone comprise 7% of lower extremity ulcers[8]. A combination of venous, arterial and diabetic disease, without any predominance, has been observed in 11% of ulcers[8]. Other rarer single causes of leg ulcers are shown in Table 1.

The costs associated with venous leg ulcers are enormous and include not only financial, but also social and psychological burdens[5]. Wood and Margolis reported that the cost of healing one leg ulcer varies from US$784 to US$6449[9], while Olin and colleagues reported that the mean cost of healing a venous ulcer was US$9685[10]. Home health care, hospitalization and home dressing changes accounted for 48%, 25% and 21% of the total cost, respectively. Studies evaluating the cost-effectiveness of different treatment options using a standardized outcome are needed[11]. Accurate diagnosis of ulcer etiology by history, physical examination and vascular tests is essential to achieve successful outcomes.

HISTORY AND PHYSICAL EXAMINATION

A detailed history and physical examination are essential in determining the cause of leg ulceration (Table 1 and Figure 1).

Venous ulcers

Patients with venous ulcers frequently complain of swelling and aching discomfort of the legs[12]. Symptoms typically increase when the patient is standing or walking and at the end of the day and decrease or are relieved with elevation of the leg[12,13]. Other symptoms include leg tiredness, itching, burning and throbbing sensations[12]. There may be a history of deep vein thrombosis, trauma or surgery to the affected leg or of multiple pregnancies[1,3]. Less frequently patients may have a history of obesity and congestive heart failure[12,14]. On physical examination venous ulcers tend to be located between the malleolus and the lower calf, an area called the gaiter area (Figure 2)[1,15]. Venous ulcers are usually shallow with irregular margins. Size is variable, but these wounds may be very large.

Table 1 Causes of leg ulcers

Vascular diseases	*Hematologic diseases*	*Infection*
Venous	Red blood cell disorders	Bacterial
Arterial	Sickle cell anemia	Furuncle
Atherosclerosis	Hereditary spherocytosis	Ecthyma
Thromboangiitis obliterans	Thalassemia	Ecthyma gangrenosum
Arteriovenous malformation	Polycythemia rubra vera	Septic emboli
Cholesterol embolism	White blood cell disorders	Gram-negative infections
Vasculitis	Leukemia	Anaerobic infections
Small vessel	Dysproteinemias	Mycobacterial
Hypersensitivity vasculitis	Cryoglobulinemia	(typical and atypical)
Rheumatoid arthritis	Cold agglutinin disease	Spirochetal
Lupus erythematosus	Macroglobulinemia	Fungal
Scleroderma	*Trauma*	Majocchi's granuloma
Sjögren's syndrome	Pressure	Deep fungal infections
Behçet's disease	Cold injury (frostbite, pernio)	Protozoal
Atrophie blanche	Radiation dermatitis	Leishmania
Medium and large vessel	Burns (thermal, chemical)	Infestations and bites
Polyarteritis nodosa	Factitia	*Panniculitis*
Nodular vasculitis	*Neoplastic diseases*	Weber–Christian disease
Wegener's granulomatosis	Epitheliomas	Pancreatic fat necrosis
Lymphatics	Squamous cell carcinoma	Necrobiosis lipoidica
Lymphedema	Basal cell carcinoma	
Neuropathic diseases	Sarcoma (e.g. Kaposi's sarcoma)	*Pyoderma gangrenosum*
Diabetes	Lymphoproliferative	
Tabes dorsalis	Lymphoma	
Syringomyelia	Cutaneous T cell lymphoma	
Metabolic diseases	Metastatic tumors	
Diabetes		
Gout		
Prolidase deficiency		
Gaucher's disease		

Reproduced by permission of Mosby Inc., from Phillips TJ, Dover JS. Leg ulcers. *J Am Acad Dermatol* 1991;25:965–87

The ulcer bed is characterized by the presence of granulation tissue or fibrinous material (Figure 3)[15,16]. Moderate to heavy exudate may be present. The surrounding skin may have red-brown hemosiderin pigmentation (Figure 4)[15,16]. Eczematous changes such as erythema, scaling, pruritus and weeping are common[15]. Periwound skin can be indurated, shiny, fibrotic and bound-down, a clinical sign called lipodermatosclerosis (Figure 3). Lipodermatosclerosis tends to occur around the ankles, but it may involve extensive areas of the leg, giving it the so-called 'inverted champagne bottle' appearance (Figure 5)[15]. Attempts to pinch the tissue between the thumb and forefinger illustrate the thickened nature of this skin (Figure 3). Edema of the lower limbs and varicosities may frequently be present.

Nelzen and co-workers reviewed the value of the classical signs in venous ulcer diagnosis (gaiter localization, varicose veins, eczema, pigmentation, induration and edema). They found that the predictive value did not exceed 0.74 for a single clinical sign and that a combination of signs did not increase the predictive value[1]. Therefore up to 26% of patients with leg ulcers secondary to venous insufficiency may have a different clinical presentation, and confirmatory studies are required.

Arterial ulcers

Patients with arterial ulcer complain of pain in the legs that is exacerbated by elevation or exertion and is relieved by dependency and

Figure 1   Ulcer management and evaluation

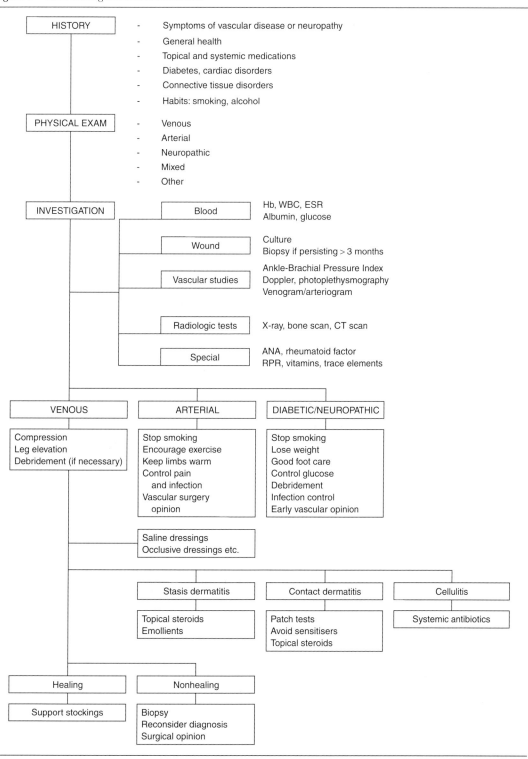

Hb, hemoglobin; WBC, white blood cell count; ESR, erythrocyte sedimentation rate; ANA, antinuclear antibodies; RPR, rapid plasma reagin. Reproduced by permission of Mosby Inc., from Phillips TJ, Dover JS. Leg ulcers. *J Am Acad Dermatol* 1991;25:965–87

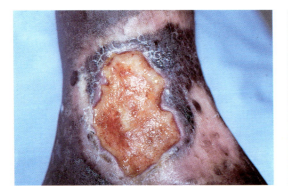

Figure 2   Venous ulcer in the typical area between the malleolus and lower calf. Ulcer edges are shallow with irregular margins. Abundant fibrinous material is observed over the ulcer surface and surrounding shiny, indurated skin

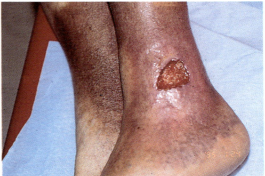

Figure 4   Venous ulcer on the gaiter area surrounded by shiny indurated tissue and marked hemosiderin deposition

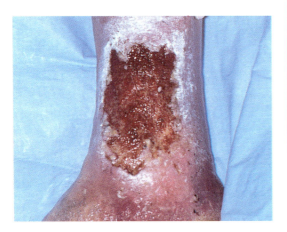

Figure 3   Venous ulcer on the gaiter area with surrounding shiny, indurated skin. There is inability to pinch tissue between the thumb and forefinger in lipo-dermatosclerosis tissue. Zinc oxide was applied to the periwound area to prevent maceration

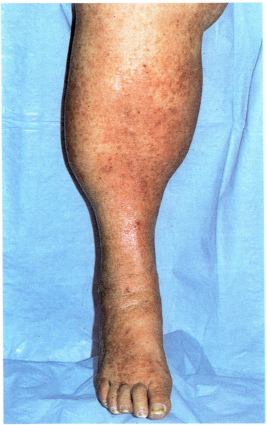

Figure 5   Leg with 'inverted champagne bottle' appearance

rest. These ulcers usually develop slowly and they characteristically affect patients older than 45 years[15]. Patients may have a history of smoking, diabetes mellitus, hyperlipidemia, or hypertension[17]. On physical examination the ulcers are usually distal and located on bony prominences. They are often sharply demarcated and have a 'punched out' appearance with a dry gray to black wound bed (Figure 6). The wound may be covered with necrotic debris and granulation tissue is often absent. The surrounding skin may have changes associated with diminished blood flow such as hair loss, shiny atrophic skin and thickened nails. The foot may be cold to the touch and peripheral pulses may be poor or

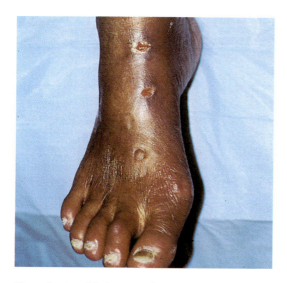

Figure 6   Arterial ulcer over dorsum of the foot

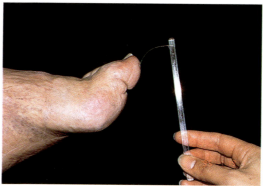

Figure 8   Use of Semmes Weinstein monofilament to evaluate pressure sensation. The monofilament is pressed against the skin with enough pressure to bend the filament

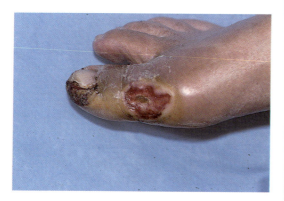

Figure 7   Neuropathic ulcer over first metatarsal

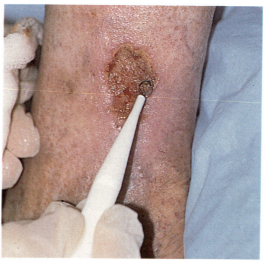

Figure 9   Debridement of an ulcer using a curette

absent. Capillary refilling time may be prolonged (more than 4 seconds). Pallor upon 45° elevation of the leg followed by redness on dependency is also suggestive of arterial disease. To test this, the leg should be elevated for at least 30 seconds. After the leg is made dependent the time until the skin color returns to normal and rubor develops should be measured. Pallor lasting 60 seconds and rubor can be correlated with a blood flow capacity of less than 10% of normal[17].

Neuropathic ulcers

Neuropathic ulcers result from repetitive trauma to pressure bearing areas including

the heels, toes and plantar metatarsal heads. The neuropathy is a chronic progressive condition that includes three components: sensory, motor and autonomic[18]. Sensory neuropathy allows painless trauma and patients may complain of tingling and burning sensations on the feet, that may increase at night and diminish with exercise[15,18]. Autonomic neuropathy leads to decreased perspiration, consequently patients also complain of dry and cracked skin[15,18]. Motor neuropathy progressively causes muscle atrophy and foot deformity leading to the development of new pressure areas or uneven distribution of pressure. On physical examination muscular atrophy and foot deformities such as hammer toes and prominent metatarsal heads may be seen[18]. Callosities on the plantar surface of the foot indicate areas of increased plantar pressure, which are areas at risk for ulceration. There is usually a callus surrounding the wound (Figure 7).

INVESTIGATIONS

Figure 1 provides information regarding the evaluation and management of ulcers. Routine laboratory tests include a complete blood count and serum glucose measurement to exclude significant hematologic diseases or diabetes mellitus[15]. Erythrocyte sedimentation rate is a helpful tool to screen for osteomyelitis, vasculitis or a connective tissue disorder[15]. When a connective tissue disorder or hypercoagulable state is suspected, screening for antinuclear antibodies, anticardiolipin antibodies, lupus anticoagulant, rheumatoid factor, rapid plasma reagin, antithrombin 3, proteins C and S, cryoglobulins, cryofibrinogen and hepatitis antibodies may be helpful. In patients with chronic venous ulcers and a history of thrombosis, activated prothrombin gene mutation and factor V Leiden should be tested[19]. If this test is positive, such a patient should be treated with anticoagulant to prevent further thrombosis and further damage to the venous system[19].

Elderly patients are at high risk of under nutrition, thus in this population serum albumin and/or transferrin levels should be performed to rule out protein deficiency. Similarly, patients with chronic leg ulcers may show lower serum levels of vitamins A and E and zinc when compared with a control population[20]. Deficiencies of vitamin C and iron have also been reported in patients with venous ulcers[21,22]. However, there are few prospective studies examining the role of vitamin and trace element supplementation on the healing rates of chronic venous ulcers[23]. Measurements of vitamin levels are not widely available and they are not currently recommended. Wound cultures may be taken at baseline, preferably by curetting or by biopsying the wound bed[15].

Vascular studies are important because patients with classical clinical signs for venous disease may have mixed venous/arterial disease[1]. Similarly, patients with neuropathic diabetic ulcers may have arterial compromise and some of them will require revascularization procedures to achieve healing. Screening for peripheral vascular disease should be performed in all patients presenting with leg ulcers. A simple objective test that can be performed in the physician's office is the ankle brachial pressure index (ABI). The ABI is the ratio of systolic pressure between the ankle and the arm in the supine position using 8 MHz Doppler ultrasonography; an ABI of around 1.0 is considered normal[8]. Patients with moderate to severe arterial disease will have an ABI of less than 0.7. These patients should be referred for vascular surgical assessment for possible arterial reconstruction[15].

Patients with diabetes are prone to calcification and decreased elasticity of the vessel walls, making the lower extremity pressures artificially elevated. In these patients the ABI is not a reliable test and to effectively identify arterial disease Doppler waveform analysis, digital (toe) pressures and arteriography are recommended[24].

The extent of the venous disease should be determined. When venous ulcers are due to limited superficial vein disease, stripping the affected veins may prevent ulcer recurrence[25,26]. Doppler ultrasonography is the cheapest and simplest test to evaluate venous insufficiency, but it may not differentiate between superficial and deep venous varieties[27]. Another technique is photoplethysmography, which assesses variations in light skin absorption by hemoglobin in dermal venous plexuses. Photoplethysmography is useful in identifying venous disease and differentiating between superficial and deep vein incompetence[15]. High-resolution duplex imaging is the accepted standard technique for venous system

Table 2 Advantages and disadvantages of compression therapy

Type	Advantages	Disadvantages
Elastic wrap	Inexpensive; can be reused. New bandages maintain compression up to 20 mmHg. Can be washed	Difficult to apply correctly. Loses elasticity. Does not maintain compression after several washes
Elastic adherent wrap	Maintains compression	Expensive
Unna's boot	Protects against trauma. Provides calf pump support. 30 mmHg compression when used with elastic bandage	Contact dermatitis, skin maceration. Gangrene can occur if applied to arterially compromised limb. Does not control heavy drainage
Four-layer bandage	Provides graduated compression – 40 mmHg at the medial malleolus and 17 mmHg below the knee. Maintains compression; comfortable, controls heavy drainage. Needs less frequent changes; can be left for seven days	Has to be applied by well-trained physicians or nurses. Bulky appearance, can be difficult to fit shoes
Compression pumps	Enhances fibrinolytic activity. Improves venous and lymphatic flow. Useful for elderly and sedentary patients; multichambered compression garments have better results (milking effect)	Expensive. Time consuming. No longer covered by Medicare
Orthotic devices circaid	Comfortable, easy to use. Sustained compression	Expensive, bulky appearance. Compliance
Support stocking	Permits frequent changes. Available with different grades of pressure	Difficult to put on, expensive, needs to be replaced every 6 months. The use of rubber gloves gives a better grip; zipper in the back facilitates application

Table reproduced with permission from Lopez AP, Bazerbashi A, Choucair M, McNeil J, Phillips TJ. The role of sustained compression in the treatment of venous ulcers. Poster presented at the Symposium on Advanced Wound Care in New Orleans, LA, April 16, 1997

evaluation of patients with venous ulcers. This system carefully differentiates between deep and superficial venous reflux and accurately identifies sites of venous reflux[27].

X-ray examination of the leg is indicated in chronic ulcers and diabetic patients to rule out osteomyelitis. Further studies such as a bone scan and bone biopsy may be considered if the X-rays are negative but the clinical presentation suggests bone infection[15].

Chronic oozing, scaling and itching on the ulcer or periwound area suggest contact dermatitis and if the causal agent is not easily identified, patch testing should be performed[15].

In ulcers that fail to improve after 3 months of appropriate treatment an excisional biopsy or punch biopsy from the edge of the ulcer is recommended to rule out malignancy, vasculitis and more uncommon causes of ulceration[15].

A nylon monofilament can help to identify diabetes patients at risk for ulceration[28]. The American Diabetic Association recommends use of the Semmes Weinstein monofilament to test pressure sensation at least once a year. The monofilament is pressed against the skin of the foot until buckling occurs (Figure 8). Measurements should be taken at ten different sites on the limb, including the leg, ankle, dorsal foot, plantar toes, metatarsal heads, instep and heel[29]. A failure to feel the monofilament at four different sites indicates loss of protective sensation.

MANAGEMENT OF LEG ULCERS

Management of patients with leg ulcers includes the evaluation and therapy of associated medical problems. This may often require a multidisciplinary team. The gold standard in the management of venous ulcers is the use of compression to reverse the effects of venous hypertension. In the case of arterial ulcers the primary goal is to increase the blood supply to the compromised area and in neuropathic ulcers, pressure relief, aggressive ulcer debridement, infection control, preventive measures and patient education are the important measures.

Compression

The first line of treatment for venous ulcers is compression, through which distended superficial veins are reduced, and by reducing the vessel area incompetent valves become competent. Compression also assists the calf muscle pump, reducing the venous pressure, increasing blood flow and thereby reducing edema[30]. Compression may be delivered using graduated compression stockings, elastic and inelastic bandages, orthotic devices and compression pumps (Table 2). The use of high compression bandaging (elastic bandages) significantly increases the odds of healing when compared to low compression bandaging[31]. Similarly, multi-layer high compression bandages seem to be more effective than single layer bandages. Compression bandages should be applied by experienced nurses in order to avoid inappropriate and varying pressures. Arterial disease should be ruled out before the application of high compression regimens[31]. Compression stockings are fitted individually and four classes are available according to the pressure delivered[32]. Class I stockings deliver 20 to 30 mmHg of pressure and are recommended for mild varicosities, edema, leg fatigue and heaviness. They are also useful during pregnancy and as thromboembolism prophylaxis. Class II (30–40 mmHg pressure) is indicated in venous insufficiency and after sclerotherapy or varicose surgery[33]. Class III delivers 40 to 50 mm and Class IV delivers more than 50 mmHg pressure. These are used in the presence of lymphedema.

Debridement

Debridement involves the removal of devitalized tissue and fibrinous material to promote formation of granulation tissue and epithelialization[34,35]. There are several methods of debridement that may be used alone or in combination. Autolytic debridement involves the use of moisture retentive dressings that enhance the function of natural proteinases. Enzymatic preparations are used for chemical debridement. Mechanical debridement may involve the use of wet to dry – or preferably wet to moist – dressings, wound irrigation, hydrotherapy and the use of dextranomers. Surgical debridement involves the use of sharp instruments such as curette, scalpel, forceps or scissors under local or general anesthesia (Figure 9).

Surgical debridement is crucial in the management of neuropathic ulcers. The use of scalpel or scissors is recommended to remove the surrounding callus and devitalized material. Shaving thin layers of hyperkeratotic tissue around the ulcers is recommended to avoid bacterial invasion to deep tissues and unnecessary bleeding[35]. Local analgesia is usually not required but should be used as needed[18]. The clinician should be familiar with the anatomy of the wound area and decide when the patient needs to be debrided by a plastic surgeon.

Aggressive debridement is usually not needed for venous ulcers, and is not recommended for arterial ulcers covered by a dry eschar[35]. These patients may have not enough blood supply to heal the wound created after debridement[35,36].

Wound dressings and topicals antiseptics

There is a wide variety of dressings, the selection of which depends upon their clinical properties, cost and availability. In acute wounds a moist environment accelerates wound resurfacing[37]. Although in chronic wounds the data are less clear, moisture retentive dressings stimulate autolytic wound debridement and formation of granulation tissue, reducing pain and infection rates[38]. Dressings should be selected according to the characteristics of the wound (clean or not), surrounding skin (presence of maceration), amount of exudate, ulcer depth, cost, presence of odor and patient compliance (Table 3). Hydrocolloids and hydrogels are preferred for mild to moderate drainage and painful ulcers. These may cause maceration that may be minimized by the use of zinc oxide paste on the periwound skin (Figure 3). Films are helpful for acute wounds with minimal or no drainage. Alginates are indicated in highly exudative ulcers. Dressing changes should be minimized to avoid disruption of newly epithelialized areas.

Topical antiseptic agents are cytotoxic *in vitro* and potentially sensitizing[39,40]. The use of hexachlorophene, benzalkonium chloride, chlorhexidine, gentian violet and alcohol should be discouraged on open wounds. Hydrogen peroxide has a transient antimicrobial activity and although toxic for fibroblasts *in vitro* did not impair wound healing *in vivo*[37,41]. Ethanoic (acetic) acid is very useful for the treatment of ulcers colonized with

Pseudomonas aeruginosa. However, in concentrations of 0.25% it impairs wound healing when compared with normal saline treated wounds[41]. Cadexomer iodine is an antiseptic that releases iodine at low concentrations which do not appear to be toxic *in vivo*[42–44]. Cadexomer iodine appears to be a safe alternative to hydrocolloids and paraffin gauze dressings in the treatment of venous leg ulcers, especially for highly exudative wounds[45,46].

The use of topical antibiotics should be limited in chronic wounds[47]. Patients with leg ulcers are highly prone to develop contact dermatitis, and topical antibiotics such as neomycin, gentamicin and bacitracin are common sensitizing agents[48]. Anaphylactic reactions to topical bacitracin and combinations of bacitracin/polymyxin ointments have been described[49–51]. Recently the use of metronidazole gel on exudative ulcers with unpleasant odors has been suggested, but safety and effectiveness studies are not available. Topical mupirocin, silvadene and erythromycin seem to be safe, although sensitization to these agents has also been reported[52]. In general, topical antibiotics should be avoided.

Table 3 Categories of wound dressing

Product	Advantages	Disadvantages
Films	Transparent, adherent; form a bacterial barrier	Fluid collection; can be difficult to apply; possibility of stripping away newly formed epithelium on removal (except Omiderm); not ideal for large amounts of exudate
Hydrogels	Comfortable, soothing; absorbent desloughing agents; semi-transparent	Non-adherent; maceration of skin around ulcer; cost
Hydrocolloids	Easy to use; cost-effective; promote granulation tissue; debride wounds	Unpleasant odor; yellow-brown, gel-like fluid drainage; difficult to use in cavities; can stimulate excess granulation tissue
Polysaccharides	Absorbent; antiseptic; desloughing	Difficult to handle; can dry out the wound bed; difficult to remove
Alginates	Absorbent; useful in sinuses; reduce frequency of dressing changes; hemostatic properties	Gel may have unpleasant odor; frequency of dressing change if wound is moist; not useful for dry wounds; require secondary dressings
Foam dressings	Absorbent; moist healing environment; conform to body contours	Can adhere to wounds if exudate dries; opaque; require secondary dressing
Laminates	Absorbent; conform to body contours	Difficult to apply; contain silicone

Reproduced with modification with permission of Health Management Publications, Inc., Wayne PA, from Choucair M, Phillips TJ. *Wounds* 1996;8:165–72

Growth factors

Growth factors influence cell growth, differentiation and the metabolism of cells participating in the wound healing process. Recombinant platelet-derived growth factor (PDGF) is the first growth factor that has been shown to be effective for the treatment of diabetic leg ulcers[53]. Other recombinant products such as epidermal growth factor (EGF), insulin-like growth factor (IGF) and fibroblast growth factor (FGF) have not shown clear benefit[54]. PDGF recruits and stimulates the proliferation of neutrophils, macrophages, fibroblasts and smooth muscle cells. It also stimulates the synthesis of collagen and extracellular matrix proteins by fibroblasts, and enhances angiogenesis and the formation of granulation tissue[55].

Topical recombinant PDGF or becaplermin hydrogel (REGRANEX®, Ortho-McNeil Pharmaceutical, Raritan, NJ) has been approved by the FDA for the treatment of lower extremity diabetic ulcers in the USA. Multicenter, double blind, placebo-controlled studies have shown increased wound closure of chronic diabetic ulcers (of more than 8 weeks' duration) after 20 weeks of daily application of becaplermin gel. At week 20 48–50% of patients treated with becaplermin achieved complete healing, compared with 25–35% of patients in the placebo group[53,56]. Similarly, the becaplermin-treated group showed decreased time to achieve complete wound closure and increased median reduction in wound area when compared with the placebo group. In these studies all the patients had aggressive surgical debridement before treatment and followed good wound practices (moist environment, control of infection and pressure relief) through the study. No difference in wound closure was seen between the control and treatment groups before 8 weeks of treatment, thus response to becaplermin is only expected to occur after 8 weeks of treatment. Becaplermin appears to be a safe therapy, with similar ulcer related adverse events such as cellulitis or osteomyelitis observed in both treatment and placebo groups.

Skin grafts

Split thickness grafts should be considered for large or non-healing wounds[57]. Split thickness grafts may be performed under local, spinal or general anesthesia. Meshing of split thickness skin grafts, especially for venous ulcers, permits the drainage of wound fluid without disturbing graft adherence to the wound bed. Excision of venous ulcers with the surrounding lipodermatosclerotic tissue, followed by application of a meshed split skin graft, has shown promising results[58,59]. Schmeller and colleagues observed a healing rate of 79% in 59 patients after 3 months, and 88% of 18 patients after an average of 2 years, using a technique called shave therapy[59].

Pinch grafting involves shaving very thin, small pieces of skin from a donor site (usually the thigh) and applying them dermal side down to the wound bed[60]. The donor skin can also be harvested using a punch biopsy[61]. Although this is a time consuming procedure, it can be performed on an outpatient basis, under local anesthetic and in patients in whom medical problems contraindicate other procedures. In Sweden pinch grafting healed between 22% and 45% of venous ulcers after 12 weeks and it is recommended as a first-line skin grafting method[62,63]. Skin grafts may work not only as tissue replacement but as pharmacologic agents that naturally secrete growth factors and cytokines that provide a stimulus for healing[64].

Skin substitutes

Skin substitutes have been classified according to their cell and matrix components into epidermal grafts, dermal grafts and composite grafts[65]. Cultured epidermal grafts are derived from the patient's own skin (autografts) or from unrelated donors (allografts). They are cultivated *in vitro* following the method developed by Rheinwald and Green[66]. These grafts have been used clinically for a variety of conditions, including burns and leg ulcers. In one study cultured epidermal autografts were used in the treatment of 35 patients with venous leg ulcers, achieving complete healing in 28 (80%) of them[67]. They are commercially available but require 3 weeks for graft cultivation. Cultured epidermal allografts could be grown in advance and cryopreserved and stored, permitting immediate availability and obviating skin biopsies that are needed to produce cultured epidermal autografts[68]. Cultured epidermal allografts have been reported in uncontrolled studies to treat venous ulcers with healing rates of 60% and 71%[69,70]. Cultured epidermal allografts were compared with hydrocolloid dressings for the treatment of chronic venous ulcers and achieved more rapid healing and a greater reduction in size, but no difference in the numbers of healed ulcers, after 6 weeks of treatment[71]. Cultured epidermal allografts are not commercially available and further controlled trials are necessary to determine their utility.

A dermal substitute composed of human dermal newborn fibroblasts cultured *in vitro* on a bioabsorbable polyglactin acid mesh has been shown to accelerate the healing of diabetic ulcers[72], but has not been approved by the FDA for this indication.

A human skin equivalent, composed of cultured human neonatal foreskin keratinocytes and fibroblasts cultivated in bovine type I collagen (Apligraf[TM]), has been used and approved by the FDA to treat venous ulcers[73]. This skin substitute is expensive, but may be useful for ulcers that are difficult to heal[74] and may be cost effective in these wounds.

Restoration of arterial supply

Surgical re-establishment of an adequate vascular supply is recommended whenever possible. An exercise program is recommended to help develop a collateral circulation, and stopping smoking (if necessary) is crucial for the process[15].

Pressure relief

Relief of mechanical stress on the injured extremity is essential for healing[75]. Off-loading of pressure from the ulcer site can be achieved by total contact cast, bed rest, walker, wheelchair or crutches plus surgical shoes, half shoes, customized sandals, or felted foams. Patients need to be informed about the rationale and techniques of off-loading[75], which should be continued until the wound is healed, with a gradual return to weight bearing as recommended by the American Diabetes Association to reduce the chance of recurrence. Appropriate footwear, proper nail care and regular visits to a foot care specialist are effective strategies.

Infection control

Infection is suggested by local inflammation, purulent drainage, sinus tract formation or crepitation, but hyperglycemia, fever, chills and leukocytosis may be absent in two thirds of patients with limb-threatening infection[28]. Treatment for osteomyelitis is recommended if bone is noticed on probing[28].

References

1. Nelzen O, Bergqvist D, Lindhagen A. Venous and non-venous leg ulcers: clinical history and appearance in a population study. *Br J Surg* 1994;81:182–7
2. Callam MJ, Harper DR, Dale JJ, Ruckley CV. Chronic ulcer of the leg: clinical history. *Br Med J (Clin Res Ed)* 1987;294:1389–91
3. Baker SR, Stacey MC, Jopp-McKay AG, *et al*. Epidemiology of chronic venous ulcers. *Br J Surg* 1991;78:864–7
4. Falanga V. Venous ulceration. *J Dermatol Surg Oncol* 1993;19:764–71
5. Phillips T, Stanton B, Provan A, Lew R. A study of the impact of leg ulcers on quality of life: financial, social, and psychological implications. *J Am Acad Dermatol* 1994;31:49–53
6. Callam MJ, Ruckley CV, Harper DR, Dale JJ. Chronic ulceration of the leg: extent of the problem and provision of care. *Br Med J (Clin Res Ed)* 1985;290:1855–6
7. Cornwall JV, Dore CJ, Lewis JD. Leg ulcers: epidemiology and aetiology. *Br J Surg* 1986;73:693–6

8. Nelzen O, Bergqvist D, Lindhagen A. Leg ulcer etiology – a cross sectional population study. *J Vasc Surg* 1991;14:557–64

9. Wood C, Margolis D. The cost of treated leg ulcers to complete healing using a occlusive dressing and a compression bandage. *Wounds* 1992;4:138–41

10. Olin JW, Beusterien KM, Beth Childs M, *et al.* Medical costs of treating venous stasis ulcers: evidence from a retrospective cohort study. *Vasc Med* 1999;4:1–7

11. Phillips TJ. Cost effectiveness in wound care. *Ostomy Wound Management* 1996;42:56–9, 62

12. Isaacs MN. Symptomatology of vein disease. *Dermatol Surg* 1995;21:321–3

13. Kanj L, Phillips T. Management of leg ulcers. *Fitzpatrick's J Clinical Dermatol* 1994;Sep/Oct: 52–60

14. Wound Ostomy and Continence Nurses. Patients with dermal wounds: lower extremity ulcers. *Standards of Care*. Laguna Beach, CA: WOCN, 1993:1–50

15. Phillips TJ, Dover JS. Leg ulcers [see comments]. *J Am Acad Dermatol* 1991;25:965–87

16. McGuckin M, Stineman M, Goin J, Williams S. *Venous Leg Ulcer Guidelines*. Philadelphia, PA: Health Management Publication Inc., 1997

17. Friedman SA. The diagnosis and medical management of vascular ulcers. *Clin Dermatol* 1990;8:30–9

18. Browne A, Sibbald R. The diabetic neuropathic ulcer: an overview. *Ostomy Wound Management* 1999;45(Suppl 1A):6–20

19. Peus D, Heit JA, Pittelkow MR. Activated protein C resistance caused by factor V gene mutation: common coagulation defect in chronic venous leg ulcers? *J Am Acad Dermatol* 1997;36:616–20

20. Rojas AI, Phillips TJ. Patients with chronic leg ulcers show diminished levels of vitamins A and E, carotenes, and zinc. *Dermatol Surg* 1999;25:601–4

21. Ette SI, Ofodile FA, Oluwasanmi JO. Vitamins and trace element profiles in chronic leg ulcers in Nigerians. *Trop Geogr Med* 1982;34:73–5

22. Balaji P, Mosley JG. Evaluation of vascular and metabolic deficiency in patients with large leg ulcers [see comments]. *Ann R Coll Surg Engl* 1995;77:270–2

23. Wilkinson EA, Hawke CI. Does oral zinc aid the healing of chronic leg ulcers? A systematic literature review. *Arch Dermatol* 1998;134: 1556–60

24. Sykes MT, Godsey JB. Vascular evaluation of the problem diabetic foot. *Clin Podiatr Med Surg* 1998;15:49–83

25. Darke SG, Penfold C. Venous ulceration and saphenous ligation. *Eur J Vasc Surg* 1992;6:4–9

26. Akesson H. Long term clinical results following correction of incompetent superficial and perforating veins in patients with deep venous incompetence and ulcers. *Phlebology* 1993;8: 128–31

27. Goldman MP, Weiss RA, Bergan JJ. Diagnosis and treatment of varicose veins: a review. *J Am Acad Dermatol* 1994;31:393–413; quiz 414–16

28. Caputo GM, Cavanagh PR, Ulbrecht JS, *et al.* Assessment and management of foot disease in patients with diabetes. *N Engl J Med* 1994; 331:854–60

29. Miller OFI. Management of diabetic foot ulcers. *J Cutan Med Surg* 1998;3:S1–13

30. Bjellerup M. Compression treatment of ulcus venosum. Mechanisms and practical guidelines. In Waersted A, Beerman B, Westbye O, Stranberg K, eds. *Treatment of Venous Leg Ulcers*. Norway: Norwegian Medicines Control Authority, 1995:87–99

31. Fletcher A, Cullum N, Sheldon TA. A systematic review of compression treatment for venous leg ulcers [see comments]. *Br Med J* 1997;315:576–80

32. Choucair M, Phillips TJ. Compression therapy. *Dermatol Surg* 1998;24:141–8

33. Sandor A, Friedman I. The diagnosis and medical management of vascular ulcers. *Clin Dermatol* 1990;8:30–9

34. Falabella A. Debridement of wounds. *Wounds* 1998;10(Suppl C):1–8

35. Sieggreen MY, Maklebust J. Debridement: choices and challenges. *Adv Wound Care* 1997; 10:32–7

36. Skillman J. Arterial leg ulcers. In Rudolph R, Noe J, eds. *Chronic Problem Wounds*. Boston: Little, Brown, 1983:103–12

37. Eaglstein WH. Occlusive dressings. *J Dermatol Surg Oncol* 1993;19:716–20

38. Nielsen P. Hydrocolloid dressings for chronic leg ulcers. In: Waersted A, Beerman B, Westbye O, Strandberg K, eds. *Treatment of Venous Leg Ulcers*. Norway: Norwegian Medicines Control Authority, 1995:111–12

39. Bolton L, Olenizcz W, Constantine B, *et al.* Repair and antibacterial effects of topical antiseptic agents *in vivo*. In Maibach H, Lowe N, eds. *Models in Dermatology*. Karger: Basel, 1985:145–58

40. Reed BR, Clark RA. Cutaneous tissue repair: practical implications of current knowledge. II. *J Am Acad Dermatol* 1985;13:919–41

41. Lineweaver W, Howard R, Soucy D, *et al.* Topical antimicrobial toxicity. *Arch Surg* 1985;120: 267–70

42. Viljanto J. Disinfection of clinical wounds without inhibition of normal wound healing. *Arch Surg* 1980;115:253–6

43. Mertz P, Davis S, Brewer L, *et al*. Can anti-microbials be effective without impairing wound healing? The evaluation of a cadexomer iodine ointment. *Wounds* 1994;6:184–93

44. Pierard-Franchimont C, Paquet P, Arrese J, Pierard G. Healing rate and bacterial necrotizing vasculitis in venous leg ulcers. *Dermatology* 1997;194:383–7

45. Hansson C. The effects of cadexomer iodine paste in the treatment of venous leg ulcers compared with hydrocolloid dressings and paraffin gauze dressing. Cadexomer Iodine Study Group. *Int J Dermatol* 1998;37:390–6

46. Falanga V. Care of venous leg ulcers. *Ostomy Wound Manage* 1999;45:33S–43S

47. Ongenae K, Phillips T. Leg ulcer management. *Emerg Med* 1993;25:45–53

48. Fisher A. Adverse reactions to bacitracin, polymyxin and gentamicin sulfate. *Cutis* 1983; 32:510–12

49. Dasaraju P, Klotz S, Bartholomew W. Photo quiz. Contact dermatitis secondary to Neosporin ointment. *Clin Infect Dis* 1997;25:33, 145

50. Dyck E, Vadas P. Anaphylaxis to topical bacitracin. *Allergy* 1997;52:870–1

51. Phillips T, Rogers G, Kanj L. Bacitracin anaphylaxis. *J Geriatr Dermatol* 1995;3:83–5

52. Zappi E, Brancaccio R. Allergic contact dermatitis from mupirocin ointment. *J Am Acad Dermatol* 1997;36:266

53. Steed D, Group DUS. Clinical evaluation of recombinant human platelet-derived growth factor for the treatment of lower extremity diabetic ulcers. *J Vasc Surg* 1995;21:71–81

54. Steed D. The role of growth factors in wound healing. *Surg Clin North Am* 1997;77:575–86

55. LeGrand E. Preclinical promise of becaplermin (rhPDGF-BB) in wound healing. *Am J Surg* 1998;176:48S–54S

56. Wieman TJ, Smiell JM, Su Y. Efficacy and safety of a topical gel formulation of recombinant human platelet-derived growth factor-BB (becaplermin) in patients with chronic neuropathic diabetic ulcers. A phase III randomized placebo-controlled double-blind study. *Diabetes Care* 1998;21:822–7

57. Hygen J. Plastic surgery in venous leg ulcers. In Waersted A, Beerman B, Westbye O, Strandberg K, eds. *Treatment of Venous Leg Ulcers.* Norway: Norwegian Medicines Control Authority, 1995

58. Galli K, Wolf H, Paul E. Therapie des ulcus cruris venosum unter berucksichtigung neurer pathogenetischer gesichtspunkle. *Phlebology* 1992;21:183–7

59. Schmeller W, Gaber Y, Gehl H. Shave therapy is a simple, effective treatment of persistent venous ulcers. *J Am Acad Dermatol* 1998;39: 232–8

60. Reverdin J. Sur la greffe epidermique. *Arch Gen Med* 1872;19:276–303

61. Korthals Atles-Levy van Vinnighe H, Faber W, Oey H. Transplantatie van huidbiopten als hulpmiddel bij de behandeling van been ulcera. *Ned T Geneeskd* 1978;122:1401–4

62. Ahnlide I, Bjellerup M. Efficacy of pinch grafting in leg ulcers of different aetiologies. *Act Derm Venereol (Stockh)* 1997;77:144–5

63. Oien R, Hansen B, Hakansson A. Pinch grafting of leg ulcers in primary care. *Acta Derm Venereol (Stockh)* 1998;78:438–9

64. Krisner R, Falanga V, Eaglstein W. The biology of skin grafts. *Arch Dermatol* 1993;129:1204–5

65. Phillips TJ. New skin for old: developments in biological skin substitutes [editorial; comment]. *Arch Dermatol* 1998;134:344–9

66. Rheinwald J, Green H. Serial cultivation of strains of human epidermal keratinocytes: formation of keratinizing colonies from single cells. *Cell* 1975;6:331–44

67. Limova M, Mauro T. Treatment of leg ulcers with cultured epithelial autografts: treatment protocol and five year experience. *Wounds* 1995;7:170–80

68. Phillips TJ, Gilchrest BA. Cultured epidermal grafts in the treatment of leg ulcers. *Adv Dermatol* 1990;5:33–48

69. De Luca M, Albanese E, Cancedda R, *et al*. Treatment of leg ulcers with cryopreserved allogenic cultured epithelium. *Arch Dermatol* 1992;128:633–8

70. Phillips TJ, Kehinde O, Green H, Gilchrest BA. Treatment of skin ulcers with cultured epidermal allografts. *J Am Acad Dermatol* 1989; 21:191–9

71. Teepe RG, Roseeuw DI, Hermans J, *et al*. Randomized trial comparing cryopreserved cultured epidermal allografts with hydrocolloid dressings in healing chronic venous ulcers. *J Am Acad Dermatol* 1993;29:982–8

72. Gentzkow GD, Jensen JL, Pollak RA, *et al*. Improved healing of diabetic foot ulcers after grafting with a living human dermal replacement. *Wounds* 1999;11:77–84

73. Falanga V, Margolis D, Alvarez O, *et al*. Rapid healing of venous ulcers and lack of clinical rejection with an allogeneic cultured human skin equivalent. Human Skin Equivalent Investigators Group [see comments]. *Arch Dermatol* 1998;134:293–300

74. Falanga V, Sabolinski M. A bilayered living skin construct (Apligraf) accelerates complete closure of hard-to-heal venous ulcers. *Wound Rep Reg* 1999;7:201–7

75. American Diabetes Association. Consensus development conference on diabetic foot wound care. *Diabetes Care* 1999;22:1354–60

Dermal manifestations of diabetes 11

R. A. Norman and R. Townsend

INTRODUCTION

Diabetes is a disease that has a huge impact on Western culture. It is estimated to account for 15% of all health care costs in the US[1]. It has been implicated as the chief cause of non-traumatic lower extremity amputations, 35% of new cases of end-stage renal disease, and a significant amount of cardiovascular disease. It has been said that the skin of all diabetic patients is affected in one way or another[2]. The elderly population is affected to a greater extent than younger people. Given that as many as 11–16 million people are affected with diabetes[2,3], the tremendous impact of the cutaneous manifestations of diabetes is obvious. The pathogenesis of these skin diseases is becoming clearer as more research is conducted. Even without that knowledge it is clear that some disorders are characteristically associated with diabetes. For example, diabetic bullae, the syndrome of waxy skin and limited joint mobility, and diabetic dermopathy are virtually pathognomonic[4].

Disorders of the diabetic skin that contribute to its pathology include microangiopathy and infection, as well as metabolic disturbances of the tissue[5]. These problems cause disease in other parts of the body as well. Consequently, it is important to understand the dermal manifestations of diabetes so one can effectively manage these sometimes common comorbidities. To this end, an outline of the more common dermal manifestations of diabetes follows; however this is not an exhaustive list, and much remains to be understood about the disease.

NECROBIOSIS LIPOIDICA DIABETICORUM

Necrobiosis lipoidica diabeticorum (NLD) (Figure 1) is not exclusive to diabetes; it is relatively rare, with an incidence of 0.7% in diabetics[6]. NLD has a greater incidence in women, and is four times more common in whites[7]. Although the average age of those affected is 34 years, there is a predominance of presentation in the young[4]. One paper reports that at the time of diagnosis, two-thirds of patients will have diabetes, and all but 10% of the rest will develop it within five years. The remainder will have an abnormal glucose tolerance test, or a first-degree relative with diabetes[3].

There are a number of potential causes associated with the disorder. Since a patient can have normal HbA1C levels, hyperglycemia is not necessarily a prerequisite for the disorder[7]. However, it does increase the chances of getting it. Antibodies and C3 have been found at the dermal/epidermal junction, which suggests a vasculitis, but other features of a leukocytoclastic vasculitis are not found[8]. In addition, Jelinek gives a list of potential causes including microangiopathy, alteration of the microcirculation, obliterative endarteritis, immune-mediated vasculitis, delayed hypersensitivity, non-enzymatic glycosylation, collagen defects, trauma, platelet aggregation, neutrophil mobility defects and vascular insufficiency[4].

Initially NLD presents as an erythematous, non-scaly plaque on the pretibial and malleolar areas of the legs[4,7]. Eventually these areas enlarge and coalesce into larger plaques that then develop yellow, atrophic centers with irregular borders that slowly enlarge[4]. The atrophy extends down into the dermis. Additionally, there are prominent telangiectasias, and approximately one-third of the lesions ulcerate. Slightly more than half the patients diagnosed with NLD have associated retinopathy and other signs of microvascular compromise[7].

Diagnosis is usually made clinically, but a biopsy can be performed. The biopsy will show an atrophic epidermis with superficial and deep granulomas. The dermis will show necrobiosis, or collagen degeneration with an absence of elastic tissue. The yellow color could be secondary to lipid deposits or deposition of β-carotene. Mucin deposits are absent. The differential diagnosis includes diseases such as sarcoidosis, granuloma annulare, lichen sclerosis, or stasis dermatitis[7].

The time required to see improvement varies from 3 to 4 years and spontaneous resolution is noted in one case in five[9]. The mainstay of treatment is tight diabetic control. Additionally topical and/or injected corticosteroids are indicated. Intralesional injection of 0.1 ml triamcinolone 2.5–10 mg/ml every 2–4 weeks has been found to be effective in severe cases[7]. Some have found aspirin in combination with dipyridamole, which modifies platelet aggregation, to be effective[10,11], while pentoxifylline has been found to be effective in others[12]. Probably the most effective treatment involves the use of a five-week course of systemic steroids. In one study six patients, four of whom were diabetic, had complete resolution. Metabolic control of their diabetes was achieved using oral hypoglycemics or insulin[13].

GRANULOMA ANNULARE

The cause of granuloma annulare (GA) is unknown. It is a benign condition that has several clinical forms[4,7], the classic type being the most common. The less common forms include generalized, multiple, perforating and subcutaneous forms[4]. This condition has lesions similar to those of NLD without the atrophic center. Lesions are common over trauma areas such as the dorsum of the hand and elbows[7]. They begin as papules and expand into annular borders with central areas of hyperpigmentation[14]. There are few other symptoms[4].

The histology of the lesion includes localized necrobiosis of collagen in the upper and mid-dermis with abundant mucin. Lesions should heal without scarring[7]. Collagen degeneration is localized with histiocytic pallisaded collagen bundles[4].

There are several forms of treatment, one of which uses liquid nitrogen to ablate the annular borders of the lesion. Intralesional injection of steroids has been tried with some efficacy[7] and one paper reported satisfactory results with isotretinoin[15]. Finally, PUVA therapy has been used successfully in some cases[16]. The therapy should probably be guided by patient preference and response to initial treatments.

DIABETIC DERMOPATHY

Diabetic dermopathy (DD) (Figure 2) has been called one of the most common skin signs of diabetes, though it can be seen in non-diabetics as well. It is more common in men with diabetes who are older than sixty[7]. The exact cause of this disorder is unknown. Some theories about the pathogenesis include post-traumatic atrophy due to a thermal or mechanical insult, or post-inflammatory hyperpigmentation in poorly vascularized skin[7,9]. There is little evidence of angiopathy or its relationship to other diabetic angiopathies. However, its incidence does correlate well with the severity of diabetes[4]. One author observed that in patients with four or more lesions, DD correlates highly with normal patients who will get diabetes, and is highly correlated with retinovascular disease in those that do have diabetes[17].

DD begins as pink patches approximately 0.5 to 1 cm in diameter on the pretibial and lateral leg areas. Eventually they become hyperpigmented brown papules with a fine scale and surface atrophy. They are round to oval, circumscribed, shallow, bilateral and usually not symmetrical. They finally heal forming scars[4,7,9]. Histologically, they display evidence of surface atrophy with thickened, small superficial blood vessels. These vessels eventually hemorrhage and leave hemosidirin deposits which give the lesions their characteristic brown color. Edema of the epidermis and papillary dermis, with a mild lymphocytic infiltrate, has also been observed[7,18]. These lesions may be differentiated from lesions that appear to be similar by observing localization, evidence of peripheral vascular disease, or presence of purpura[4]. Similar-looking lesions can be found in traumatic scars, stasis dermatitis, pigmentary purpuras and early NLD[7].

Treatment is not necessary since these lesions resolve spontaneously[7].

DIABETIC THICK SKIN

Some clinicians have noted that patients with diabetes mellitus have thicker skin than those without. This phenomenon has been studied using ultrasound to determine the difference between subjects and controls[9,19,20].

Three aspects of skin changes in this group of patients were demonstrated; one group had clinically inapparent, but measurable changes; another group had clinically apparent changes ranging from pebbled skin to scleroderma-like changes; and an infrequent syndrome of scleredema developed in some that resulted in marked thickening of the skin of the upper back[9]. Support for this comes from the finding that patients with type I diabetes, even those without clinical evidence of skin thickening, showed changes when biopsies were examined and compared with controls[19]. Hundley and Walter demonstrated that increased skin thickness was not universal in all diabetics, nor that it was necessarily even over all parts of the body[20]. It has also been shown that thickening occurs predominantly on the extremities[9].

Histologically there are large disorganized bundles of collagen separated by clear spaces and small amounts of acid mucopolysaccharides. Electron microscopy has demonstrated a thickened basement membrane as in scleroderma, but large collagen fibers – not in a bimodal pattern – predominate, unlike the situation in scleroderma[19].

There is no treatment for this condition.

DIABETIC SCLEREDEMA

Two studies have described the incidence of this disorder (Figure 3). In one study, at a veterans administration medical center, 2.5% of the diabetic patients were described as having diabetic scleredema[21]. The incidence has been found to be as high as 14% in a population at a Kuwait hospital[22]. It is found predominantly in obese, insulin-dependent, middle-aged males who have microvascular complications and whose diabetes is poorly controlled[9,21].

There are two forms of this disorder. The classic form is scleredema adultorum of Buschke that commonly affects non-diabetic children, and is heralded by an acute streptococcal infection[7,21]. The other form is found in diabetics[7].

Symptoms include a taut thickening of the skin of the upper back, neck and shoulders with extension to the face, arms, chest and abdomen in some. This can include a hardened, non-pitted, shiny surface without markings or wrinkles. Additionally, the skin cannot be pressed into folds. The diabetic form tends to involve a greater surface area than the non-diabetic form[4,7].

In order to properly diagnose this condition laboratory tests to screen for scleroderma and dermatomyositis should be included. Additionally, ASO titers, immunoglobulin titers (to rule out gammopathies) and deep wedge biopsies should be done to aid in diagnosis[7]. Histologically, the tissue samples should have large collagen bundles separated by wide clear spaces. There might be an increased number of mast cells in the section[23].

Better control of the patient's diabetes offers the only chance of alleviating this condition, but results are generally poor and no treatment is very effective[7,9]; however, most lesions resolve spontaneously[4].

DIABETIC THICK SKIN OF THE FINGERS

Although it may seem that this disorder has many characteristics in common with diabetic thick skin, it does have several features that set it apart. For instance, this disorder is found predominantly in the young, though it can affect adults, in whom the disorder is less severe[24]. The condition has been reported in as many as 50% of adolescent diabetic patients who have had their illness more than five years[25].

The pathology of the disorder involves a stiffening of the collagen and periarticular tissues. However the joint itself is not directly involved[4]. Some authors have suggested that this change may actually represent accelerated aging of the collagen. They also noticed an association with microvascular complications such as retinopathy and nephropathy[7]. Others felt that thick skin of the hand foretold microvascular complications later in life, especially in the young[25].

Symptoms of this disorder are much as they sound. Generally, the appearance is that of scleroderma without Raynaud's[26]. More specifically, the diabetic hand syndrome consists of thickened skin over the dorsum of the hand, and limited joint mobility, especially of the interphalangeal joints[4,27]. The joint limitation may vary from mild to contracture[28]. The stiffening usually begins at the metacarpophalangeal and proximal interphalangeal joints of the fifth finger, and progresses to involve others[29]. This effect on the hands is usually bilateral, symmetric and painless. Initially the limitation is in passive motion, but eventually will involve active motion as well[30]. Limitation can be demonstrated by a positive 'prayer sign'. This occurs when the hands are placed palm to palm as in prayer, with a subsequent inability to straighten the fingers. However, the most accurate way to determine limitation is by the examiner's passively testing the joints[31]. Finally, since the syndrome is most often observed in children, it is important to check for growth and maturational delays which are associated with this disorder[9]. Histologic findings of note consist of a waxy thickening of the collagen fibers in affected tissues[7].

Unfortunately, treatment is generally unrewarding. The only treatment that has been shown to be effective is tight diabetic control using an insulin pump[32].

DIABETIC BULLAE

This rare disorder has only had little more than 100 cases reported in the literature (Figure 4). It is most common in patients who have long-term Type II diabetes, and who have developed peripheral neuropathy[7]. Additionally, so far, the disorder has only been described in men[4].

Lesions develop spontaneously and are not necessarily associated with trauma[7,28]. The term diabetic bullae is really a heterogeneous term that describes a spectrum of bullous lesions that appear spontaneously in diabetics[7]. There is some debate over the etiology of these bullae. Some authors feel that diabetic bullae may develop at sites of trauma even if the patients do not recall the incident[33,34], and some authors do not.

There are three types of diabetic bullae. The most common type has a non-inflammatory base, contains clear, sterile fluid, and heals without scarring[35]. Another unusual type heals with scarring, and with dystrophic epidermolysis bullosa, by forming a cleavage line below the dermo-epidermal junction by destroying the anchoring fibrils[33,36]. The third, and most unusual, type forms subepidermal bullae that mimic porphyria cutanea tarda. It occurs primarily in a photo-distribution[7]. These lesions measure about 0.5 cm to 1 cm, appear suddenly, and occur bilaterally with tense bullae primarily on the legs and feet. Occasionally they can be found on the hands as well[4]. It is important to keep in mind the differential for bullous diseases. This includes bullous impetigo, bullous pemphigoid, pemphigus vulgaris, epidermolysis bullosa acquisita, porphyria cutanea tarda, bullous erythema multiforme and insect bite reaction[2].

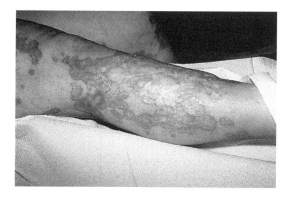

Figure 1   Necrobiosis lipoidica

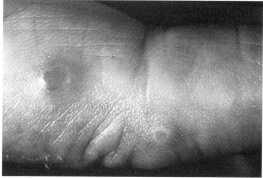

Figure 4   Diabetic bullae

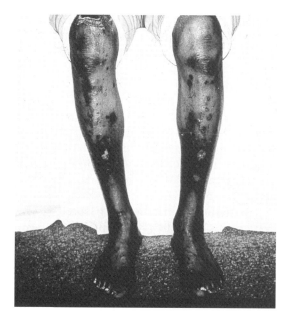

Figure 2   Diabetic dermopathy

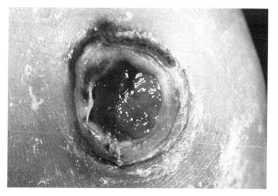

Figure 5   Mal perforans

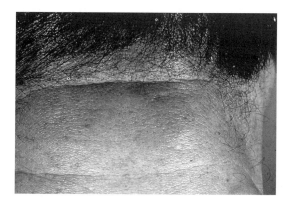

Figure 3   Scleredema diabeticorum

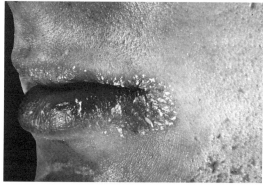

Figure 6   Angular stomatitis

Histologically these lesions usually occur intra-epidermally[35], but some have been reported as being subepidermal. However it has been pointed out that some of these reported differences could be the result of biopsies being taken at different stages of development[34].

Treatment consists of preventing infection, since these lesions generally heal spontaneously in two to five weeks[4].

ACANTHOSIS NIGRICANS

Acanthosis nigricans is a condition that can be associated with disorders of insulin resistance such as diabetes, obesity[37] and occasionally with paraneoplastic syndromes[7]. It has been reported to occur with an incidence approaching 74% in otherwise healthy obese adults[38], 66% in primary school children who weigh 200% of ideal body weight, 28% of children weighing 120% of ideal body weight, and 7.1% in an unselected population of primary school children[39]. It has also been demonstrated to occur with higher frequency in certain ethnic populations. Native Americans have an incidence of acanthosis nigricans of 54%, and it occurs at an incidence of 40% in Hispanic populations[40].

Most authors have causally linked acanthosis nigricans to pathology related to the insulin growth factor (IGF) receptors found in the epidermis[9,14]. The defect has been postulated to be related to defects in the receptor itself, postreceptor function, antibodies, or obesity[41]. Additionally, there are three lines of evidence that associate this disorder with high plasma levels of insulin. These include the finding of classic insulin receptors and IGF receptors in fibroblasts and keratinocytes in the epidermis. Second, acanthosis nigricans has been found locally at the site of injection of insulin. Finally, as previously mentioned, most of the conditions associated with the disorder have a form of insulin resistance[9].

Symptoms include velvety, hyperpigmented plaques, which are found on the flexural areas and the back of the neck. Additionally, there can be an associated papillomatosis[7]. These lesions can range from shallow to deep[9].

Histologically the lesions show marked hyperkeratosis, papillomatosis, and are mildly acanthotic[33]. Some also display atrophy and increased amounts of melanin in the basal epidermis[9,42].

There are several ways to treat this disorder. One way is to use keratolytic agents such as salicylic acid. Some success has also been obtained by the use of omega-3 fatty acids and a diet rich in fish oils. Weight control and exercise[7] are very beneficial in controlling the disorder; in all probability, a combination of these treatments with good serum glucose control will be the best approach.

DIABETIC YELLOW NAILS AND SKIN

Yellow nails and skin is a condition commonly associated with diseases such as onychomycosis and psoriasis, and with aging. However, this condition is found in as many as one-half of diabetic patients[43]. Additionally some complications of diabetes have been directly correlated to increased levels of certain non-enzymatic glycosylation end-products in skin biopsies. These include limited joint mobility[44], retinopathy[44,45], and nephropathy[44].

The pathology has been attributed to several sources, including carotemia[7], but a more probable cause is glycosylation of proteins because of poor glycemic control[8]. Glycosylation yields an end product called 2-(2-furoyl)-4(5)-(2-furanyl)-1H-imidazole, which has a yellow hue and could, therefore, contribute to the yellow color of the skin[9]. The change leaves the distal halux of the nail with a yellowish tint[43], and the yellow color of the skin is best appreciated on the palms and soles owing to the sparse number of melanocytes in these areas[9].

There is no treatment for this condition, nor has the real significance of this disorder been determined[9]. However, it seems reasonable to suppose that better serum glucose control will give rise to fewer problems.

PERFORATING DERMATOSIS

This disease is generally found in middle aged black males (Figure 5)[4]. It is worth noting

that it has been split into several subcate-
gories. Names such as Kyrle's disease, reactive
perforating folliculitis, reactive perforating
collagenosis and acquired perforating elastosis appear in the literature[7,46]. However, these
distinctions are somewhat academic and the
similarities outweigh the differences[46]. One
major association is that this disorder occurs
almost exclusively in endstage nephropathy.
The pathology behind the disorder consists
of transepidermal elimination of collagen
and elastin[46]. Additionally, one author has
implicated neutrophils in the pathologic
process.

Symptoms of perforating dermatosis
include endstage nephropathy and multiple
skin lesions. Lesions are papular, hyperkeratotic, pruritic and occasionally umbilicated.
They are usually located on the extensor surfaces of the legs. Often they coalesce into
larger plaques, but can exist in rows. Excoriation or trauma (Koebner phenomenon) can
induce them[4,7].

Histologically, the lesions are composed of
epidermis encircling a plug of degenerative
material, which has elements of collagen,
elastin, nuclear material and neutrophils in it.
As in eczema, spongiosis and acanthosis may
be seen[33].

Unfortunately, these lesions have little tendency to resolve on their own[4] and the pruri-
tis is a very difficult feature of the problem to
treat[7]. Two treatments that have some efficacy
against the lesions are UVB[7] and retinoic
acid[7,47]; topical antipruritics can be used to
treat the itching[7].

CUTANEOUS INFECTIONS

Cutaneous infection is the area of diabetic
skin disease that is most often thought about
although, in fact, well-controlled diabetics
probably are no more susceptible to infection
than the normal population. However, poor
control (especially ketoacidosis) compromises
resistance. The poorly controlled get more
severe, protracted and resistant infections[4].
Once serum glucose control is re-established,
resistance usually returns to normal[48].

Contrary to expectation, hyperglycemia
contributes little to the growth of most cutaneous organisms; indeed, topically applied
sugar and honey have actually been used in
healing ulcers of the skin[49]. A well-known
exception is *Candida*, for which there is a
direct correlation between growth and sugar
concentration in the saliva[50]. Infection is
actually one of the most important triggers of
ketoacidosis[4]. In the literature, cutaneous
infection has been associated with ketoacidosis[4], abnormal function of granulocytes[51,52],
peripheral vascular disease and sensory
impairment[4] and dry skin[4]. These problems
can occur individually, but are often found in
combination.

Candida

Candida is one organism that has a strong
relationship to increased serum sugar levels
and may be an early indicator of undiagnosed diabetes. It is commonly seen in older
patients whose diabetes is not controlled[7]. In
the young, angular stomatitis (Figure 6) is a
classic complication, and has been found to
be linearly related to the amount of sugar in
the saliva[7,50,53]. Additionally, *Candida* has been
reported to infect the hands and feet[7], but
the incidence in diabetics may not be any
higher than that in the general population[54].
On the hands it occurs as paronychia. Other
places that are commonly infected include
the web spaces of the fingers and toes. The
appearance of this infection is quite similar
to that of dermatophytes. It is distinguished
by failure to respond to medication, or culture. The final area involved is that of the
nail plates. Fortunately, the living tissue does
not appear to be involved[7,9]. Further, women
may have problems with inframammary and
vaginal infections[7,55] and men can get infections such as balanitis which can result in
phimosis[4,7].

Treatment of these infections is generally
routine. Topical antifungals and, occasionally,
systemic antifungals help the patients.
Needless to say, normalization of the blood
sugar is necessary, too[7].

Bacterial infections

Cutaneous bacterial infections in diabetics are most commonly caused by organisms such as *Staphylococcus aureus*, *Escherichia coli*, beta hemolytic streptococcus, and *Pseudomonas*. *Staphylococcus* and *Streptococcus* are implicated in infections such as impetigo, folliculitis, furuncles, carbuncles, ecthyma, cellulitus and erysipelas. The greatest complication of any of these infections in the diabetic is gangrene of the extremities. Control involves glycemic control, debridement and appropriate parenteral antibiotics[7]. Increased rates of staphylococcal infections have been demonstrated in patients using subcutaneous pumps to deliver their insulin[56,57]. Similarly, 30% of Group B streptococcal infections occur in diabetic patients[58–60], and there is a 3.2-fold increase in the relative risk for diabetics of aquiring Group A infections[61].

Pseudomonas is a potentially life threatening infection; in particular otitis externa caused by *Pseudomonas* is a serious infection in the elderly diabetic. Malignant otitis externa is characterized by discharge from the canal and severe pain. Infection progresses from a cellulitis to chondritis, to osteomyelitis, and eventually meningitis[7]. Spread through these tissue planes leaves half its victims dead. A much more common place to infect includes the toe web spaces and nails. The nail gains a green discoloration. Treatment includes diluted vinegar for superficial cutaneous infections, and debridement accompanied by an antipseudomonal antibiotic if a deeper infection occurs[9].

Nail infections in diabetics deserve special comment. While the infection itself is not life threatening, complications from the dystrophic nail can result in infection and eventual amputation. Thus, aggressive foot care is of paramount importance. Organisms to consider in nail infections include dermatophytes, *Pseudomonas aeruginosa*, *Staphylococcus aureus*, *Escherichia coli*, *Proteus mirabilis*, *Candida albicans*, and *Candida parapsilosis*[7]. Consequently, nail infections that are unresponsive to conventional treatment should be biopsied, and treatment adjusted accordingly.

Dermatophytes

These organisms are not found to infect the diabetic more than the general population[54]. As previously mentioned, they need to be treated expeditiously because of the possibility of secondary complications. Treatment includes itraconazole at 200 mg each day, for one week per month for four months; terbinafine at 250 mg per day for three months is also quite effective[9].

Erythrasma

Corynebacterium minutissimum causes tannish-red, fine scaly patches in the intertriginous zones. It can be diagnosed by its coral-red glow under a Wood's lamp. Topical or systemic erythromycin is curative[9].

Phycomycetes

This organism can be found in leg ulcers, non-healing wounds and surgical wounds, especially those not responding to treatment. Diagnosis is confirmed by culture and histological demonstration of fungal elements invading the vasculature. Characteristic findings include black crusting on the turbinates, septum and palate. Cerebral involvement occurs in two-thirds of patients. Correcting ketoacidosis is the first step in treatment, followed by debridement and intravenous amphotericin[9].

LIPODYSTROPHY LIPOHYPERTROPHY

Lipodystrophy occurs as a complication of injection, appearing as a circumscribed, depressed area at the site of injection. It used to occur more often before the introduction of purified human insulin[7]. It is probably caused by a local immune response[62].

Lipohypertrophy is a reaction that occurs locally at the site of insulin injection. It has been reported as occurring at an incidence of 14% in patients with diabetes[63] and has been attributed to a combination of local and systemic allergic reactions[2].

PERIUNGUAL TELANGIECTASIA

The periungual area is an excellent site for viewing the functional and structural changes to a diabetic patient's microcirculation. A good method is to use a small amount of mineral oil on the area, wait a few minutes for it to become translucent, and then view it with a 40x ophthalmoscope or a low power microscope. Changes are characteristic according to how long the patient has had diabetes. A newly diagnosed individual with early changes will have simple capillary loops with dilated veins. Later changes in someone who was poorly controlled, but now has excellent control, include venous tortuosity without dilatation. More extensive changes are small hemorrhages and dropout areas[9,64]. Venous dilatation has been reported in as many as 49% of diabetic patients compared with 10% of controls. It is important to recall that connective tissue diseases show periungual changes with megacapillaries, or irregularly enlarged loops[65].

ERYSIPELAS-LIKE ERYTHEMA

Although not common, a well-demarcated erythema of the lower extremities with destruction of the underlying bone, and consequent gangrene, has been reported. It is distinguished by the fact that it has no pyrexia, increased erythrocyte sedimentation rate or leukocytosis. The pathology behind the problem seems to come from a functional microangiopathy localized to an area of macrocirculatory compromise[9].

ERUPTIVE EXANTHOMAS

These lesions are characteristic of hyperlipidemic states[4]. They may result from the accumulation of foamy, or exanthoma, cells, which are macrophages that incorporate lipoproteins due to the hyperlipidemic state[66]. The lesisons are characterized by multiple, firm, yellow, waxy papules about 1–4 mm in diameter which occur on the extensor surfaces, pressure points and popliteal surfaces[67]. Sometimes they become itchy and tender and develop an erythematous halo. They have also been known to exhibit Koebner's phenomenon[68].

The only treatment includes correction of the hyperlipidemic and hyperglycemic states[67].

CALCIPHYLAXIS

This disorder is seen in middle aged to older diabetic males and it is also seen in end-stage renal disease, advanced HIV and secondary hyperparathyroidism. The etiology of the disorder is poorly understood. The lesions begin as preinfarctive, ischemic plaques, or mottled areas. They have a dusky color that ranges from erythematous to violaceous. They are exquisitely tender, and indurated. Later, bullae form as the epidermis becomes necrotic. This eventually sloughs forming an ulcer. The central area is usually black, owing to infarcted tissue. The lesions will enlarge over weeks to months. The differential diagnosis includes necrobiosis lipoidica, dystrophic calcinosis cutis, metastatic cancer, scleroderma, pyoderma gangrenosum, warfarin necrosis and hepatic necrosis. Diagnosis is made by biopsy, serum calcium, history, and parathyroid hormone level.

Treatment primarily includes debridement. It is also necessary to treat the hypercalcinosis, renal failure, hyperparathyroidism and secondary infections[69].

CONCLUSION

Diabetes is responsible for significant worldwide morbidity and enormous health care costs. Every diabetic patient has a skin malady, so one must use diagnostic acumen to provide the best care for the patients. The physician is a crucial player in the fight against diabetes and needs to be aware of the skin signs of diabetes. Many dermatological manifestations of diabetes, including diabetic dermopathy, scleredema, thick skin, bullae, and cutaneous infections can be observed if one is aware of their manifestations. In particular, the authors recommend checking the hands and feet of all diabetic patients and looking for the often destructive insults of the disease. With proper inspection and education, patients can be saved from the devastating effects of diabetes.

References

1. Javitt JC, *et al. Diabetes in America*, 2nd edn. Bethesda, MD: NIH, 1995
2. Rifkin H, Ellenberg M, eds. *Diabetes Mellitus: Theory and Practice*, 3rd edn. New Hyde Park, NY: Medical Examination Publishing Co., 1983
3. Muller SA, Winkelman RK. Necrobiosis lipoidica diabeticorum, a clinical and pathological investigation of 171 cases. *Arch Dermatol* 1966;93:272–81
4. Jelinek JE. Cutaneous manifestations of diabetes mellitus. *Int J Dermatol* 1994;33:605–17
5. Forst T, Pfutzner A, Kunt T, *et al*. Skin microcirculation in patients with type I diabetes with and without neuropathy after neurovascular stimulation. *Clin Sci* 1998;94:255–61
6. Yefimor AS, Skroboskaia NA, Shecherbak AV, *et al*. Lipoid necrobiosis in diabetes mellitus patients. *Vrach Delo* 1984;5:42–3
7. Sibald GR, *et al*. Skin and diabetes. *Endocrinol Metab Clin North Am* 1996;25:463–72
8. Dahl MV, Ullman S, Fisher I. Direct immunofluorescence of granuloma annulare and necrobiosis lipoidica. *Clin Res* 1976;24:95a
9. Electronic Textbook of Dermatology, Diabetes-Update. http://telemedicine.org/dm/dmupdate.htm
10. Heng MCY, Song MK, Heng MK. Healing of necrobiotic ulcers with antiplatelet therapy: correlation with plasma thromboxane levels. *Int J Dermatol* 1989;28:195–7
11. Quinby SR, Muller SA, Schroeter AL, *et al*. Necrobiosis diabeticorum: platelet survival and response to platelet inhibitors. *Cutis* 1989; 42:213–16
12. Noz KC, Korstanje MJ, Vermeer BJ. Ulcerating necrobiosis lipoidica effectively treated with pentoxifylline. *Clin Exp Dermatol* 1993;18:78–9
13. Petzelbauer P, Wolff K, Tappeina G. Necrobiosis lipoidica: treatment with systemic corticosteroids. *Br J Dermatol* 1992;126:542–5
14. Cruz PD. Excess insulin binding to insulin like growth factor receptors: proposed mechanism for acanthosis nigrans. *J Invest Dermatol* 1992; 98(Suppl):825–855
15. Schleicher SM, Milstein HJ, Lim SMJ, Stanton CD. Resolution of disseminated granuloma annulare with isotretinoin. *Int J Dermatol* 1992; 31:371–2
16. Kerker BJ, Huang CP, Morison WL. Photochemotherapy of generalized granuloma annulare. *Arch Dermatol* 1992;126:359–61
17. Murphy RA. Skin lesions in diabetic patients: the 'spotted leg' syndrome. *Lahey Clin Found Bull* 1965;14:10–14
18. Binkley GW, Giraldo B, Stoughton RB. Diabetic dermopathy: a clinical study. *Cutis* 1967;3:955–8
19. Hanna W, Friesen D, Bomberdier C, *et al*. Pathologic features of diabetic thick skin. *J Am Acad Dermatol* 1987;16:546–53
20 Huntley AC, Walter RM. Quantitative evaluation of skin thickness in diabetes mellitus: relationship to disease parameters. *J Med* 1990; 21:257–64
21. Cole GW, Headley J, Skowsky R. Scleredema diabeticorum: a common and distinct cutaneous manifestation of diabetes mellitus. *Diabetes Care* 1983;6:189–92
22. Monnier VM, *et al*. Relation between complications of type I diabetes mellitus and collagen-linked fluorescence. *N Engl J Med* 1986;314: 403–8
23. Cohn BA, Wheeler CE, Briggamon RA. Scleredema adultorum of Buschke and diabetes mellitus. *Arch Dermatol* 1970;101:27–35
24. Larkin JG, Frier BM. Limited mobility and Dupuytren's contracture in diabetic hypertensive and normal populations. *Br Med J* 1986; 292:1494
25. Rosenblum AL, Silverstein JH, Lezotte DC, *et al*. Limited joint mobility in childhood diabetes mellitus indicated increased risk for microvascular disease. *N Engl J Med* 1981; 305:191–4
26. Dowd PM, Gaywood IC, Kurtz AB, *et al*. Diabetic sclerodactyly. *Br J Dermatol* 1986;115:21
27. Brik R, Berant M, Verdi P. The scleroderma-like syndrome of insulin-dependent diabetes mellitus. *Diabet Metabol Rev* 1991;7:121–8
28. Huntley AC. Cutaneous manifestations of diabetes mellitus. *Dermatol Clin* 1989;7:531–46
29. Rosenbloom AL. Skeletal and joint manifestations of childhood diabetes. *Pediatr Clin North Am* 1984;31:569–89
30. Grgic A, Rosenbloom AL, Weber FT, *et al*. Joint contracture in childhood diabetes. *N Engl J Med* 1975;292:372

31. Rosenbloom AL. Limited joint mobility in insulin-dependent childhood diabetes. *Europ J Pediatr* 1990;149:380–8

32. Lieberman LS, Rosenblum AL, Riley WJ, *et al.* Reduced skin thickness with pump administration of insulin. *N Engl J Med* 1980;303:940–1

33. Parex I. Cutaneous manifestations of diabetes mellitus. *J Am Acad Dermatol* 1994;30:519–31

34. Bernstein JE. Reduced threshold to suction-induced blister formation in insulin epidermolysis bullosa without immunoreactants. *J Am Acad Dermatol* 1983;8:790–5

35. Nieboer C, Kalsbeck GL. Direct immunofluorescence studies in granuloma annulare, necrobiosis lipoidica, and granulomatosis disciforms miescher. *Dermatologia* 1979;158:427–32

36. Burnstein JE. Bullous eruptions of diabetes mellitus. *Arch Dermatol* 1979;115:324–5

37. Raevan GM. Role of insulin resistance in human disease. *Diabetes* 1988;37:1595–607

38. Hud JA Jr, *et al.* Prevalence and significance of acanthosis nigrans in an adult obese population. *Arch Dermatol* 1992;128:941–4

39. Stuart CA, Pate CJ, Peters EJ. Prevalence of acanthosis nigrans in an unselected population. *Am J Med* 1989;87:269–72

40. Bent KN, *et al.* Acanthosis nigrans as an early clinical proxy marker of increased risk of type II diabetes mellitus. *Pub Health Nurs* 1989;15:415–21

41. Rendon MI, Cruz PD, Sontheimer RD. Acanthosis nigrans: cutaneous marker of tissue resistance to insulin. *J Am Acad Dermatol* 1989;21:461–9

42. Rosenblum AL, Frais JL. Diabetes mellitus, short stature and stiff joints: a new syndrome. *Clin Res* 1974;22:92As

43. Lithner F, Hietake SO. Skeletal lesions of the foot and their relationship to cutaneous erythema with and without necrosis of the bone. *Act Med Scand* 1976;200:155–61

44. Sell DR, *et al.* Pentasidine formation in skin correlates with severity of complications in individuals with long-standing insulin dependent diabetes mellitus: decision and cost effectiveness analyses. *J Am Med Assoc* 1995;273:712–20

45. McCance DR, *et al.* Maillord reaction end products and their relation to complications in insulin dependent diabetes mellitus. *J Clin Invest* 1993;91:2470–8

46. Rapini RP. Acquired perforating dermatosis: evidence for combined transepidermal elimination of both collagen and elastic fibers. *Arch Dermatol* 1989;125:1074–8

47. Berger RS. Reactive perforating collagenosis of renal failure: diabetes responsive to topical retinoic acid. *Cutis* 1989;43:540–2

48. Edwards JE, Tillman DB, Miller ME, *et al.* Infection and diabetes mellitus. *Western J Med* 1979;130:515–21

49. Chirife J, Scarmato G, Herszag L. Scientific basis of using granulated sugar in the treatment of infected wounds. *Lancet* 1982;i:560–1

50. Knight L, Fletcher J. Growth of *Candida albicans* in saliva: stimulation by glucose associated with antibiotics, steroids, and diabetes mellitus. *J Infect Dis* 1971;123:371–7

51. Hill HR, Souls HS, Dattloff JL. Impaired leukocyte responsiveness in patients with juvenile diabetes mellitus. *Clin Immunol Immunopathol* 1974;2:395–403

52. Bagdade JD, Stewart M, Walters E. Impaired granulocyte adherence: a reversible defect in host defense in patients with poorly controlled diabetes. *Diabetes* 1978;27:677–81

53. Bartholemew GA, Rodu B, Bell DS. Oral candidiasis in patients with diabetes mellitus: a thorough analysis. *Diabetes Care* 1987;10:607–12

54. Lugo-Somonlinos A, Sanchez JL. Prevalence of dermatophytosis in patients with diabetes. *J Am Acad Dermatol* 1991;26:408–10

55. Sonck CE, Sonersalo O. The yeast flora of the anogenital area in diabetic girls. *Arch Dermatol* 1963;88:846–52

56. Chantelau E, *et al.* Acute cutaneous complications and catheter needle colonization during insulin pump treatment. *Diabetes Care* 1987;10:478–82

57. van Faasen I, Razenburg PPA, Simons-Smit AM, vander Veen EA. Carriage of *Staphylococcus aureus* and inflamed infusion sites with insulin pump therapy. *Diabetes Care* 1989;12:153–5

58. Farley MM. A population based assessment of invasive disease due to group B streptococcus in nonpregnant adults. *N Engl J Med* 1993;328:1807–11

59. Schwartz B, *et al.* Invasive group B streptococcal disease in adults: a population-based study in metropolitan Atlanta. *J Am Med Assoc* 1991;266:1112–14

60. Munoz P, *et al.* Group B streptococcus bacteremia in nonpregnant adults. *Arch Int Med* 1997;157:213–16

61. Davies HD, *et al.* Invasive group A streptococcal infections in Ontario, Canada: Ontario group A streptococcal study group. *N Engl J Med* 1996;335:547–54

62. Wright AD, Walsch CH, Fitzgerald MG, *et al.* Very pure porcine insulin in clinical practice. *Br Med J* 1979;1:25–7

63. Page MD, Bodansky HJ. Human insulin and lipoatrophy (Letter). *Diabet Med* 1992;9:779

64. Landau J, Davis E. The small blood vessels of the conjunctiva and nailbeds in diabetes mellitus. *Lancet* 1960;2:731–4

65. Grassi W, Gasparini M, Cerrini C. Nailfold computed videomicroscopy in morphofunctional assessment of diabetic microangiopathy. *Acta Diabetol Lat* 1985;22:223–8

66. Parker F, Bagdade JD, Odland GF, *et al.* Evidence for the chylomicron origin of lipids accumulating in diabetic eruptive exanthomas: a correlative lipid, biochemical, histochemical, and electron microscope study. *J Clin Invest* 1970;49:2172–87

67. Cruz PO, East C, Berstresser PR. Dermal, subcutaneous, and tendon exanthomas: diagnostic markers for specific lipoprotein disorders. *J Am Acad Dermatol* 1988;19:95–111

68. Roederer G, Xhignesser M, Davignon J. Eruptive and tuboeruptive exanthomas of the skin arising on sites of previous injury: two case reports. *J Am Med Assoc* 1988;260:1282–3

69. Fitzpatrick TB, Johnson RA, Wolff K, *et al.* *Color Atlas and Synopsis of Clinical Dermatology, Common and Serious Diseases*, 3rd edn. New York: McGraw-Hill, 1997:426–9

Index